THE SURVIVAL GUIDE TO GIVING BIRTH

WELCOMING BABIES TO THE WORLD

MAUREEN GANNON

Maureen Gannon asserts the moral right to be identified as the author of the work. The work is based on the authors many years' experience working within the profession of Midwifery. All rights are reserved.

No part of this publication may be reproduced, stored in a retrieval system or transmitted, in any form or by any means, electronic, mechanical, photocopying, recording, or otherwise, without prior permission from the publishers.

This book is sold subject to the condition that it shall not, by the way of trade or otherwise, be lent, re-sold, hired out or otherwise circulated without the publisher's prior consent in any form of binding or cover, other than that, in which it is published and without a similar condition including this condition being imposed on the subsequent purchaser

Copyright Written Work: © Maureen Gannon 2021

Copyright Cover Image: © Pen & Ink Designs 2021

Publisher: Pen & Ink Designs 2021

ISBN: 9780993112966

Dedication

To my dear children, Cheryl, Simon and Tim,

my lovely grandchildren, Paul, Miles, Niamh, Bryn and Cerys,

and my delightful great-grandchildren, Megan and Alfie.

With all my love.

CONTENTS

PREPARING FOR CONCEPTION	7
VOCABULARY OF PREGNANCY AND LABOUR	12
THE ROLE OF THE PROFESSIONALS	17
SAME-SEX PARENTING	24
SINGLE PARENTS	27
SURROGACY	30
MISCONCEPTIONS OF THE BIRTH PROCESS	32
WISE NUTRITION	37
MORNING SICKNESS	40
EXERCISE	42
PSYCHOLOGY	43
HOW THE UNBORN BABY RESPONDS TO STIMULI	48
LOW-RISK / HIGH-RISK PREGNANCY	52
TYPES OF BIRTH	54
BIRTH OPTIONS	58
CASCADE OF INTERVENTION	73
BIRTH PARTNER / COMPANION	80

CONTENTS

ROLE OF THE BIRTH PARTNER DURING BIRTH	84
BIRTH DOULA	88
PREPARING A BIRTH PLAN	90
SUGGESTIONS FOR YOUR BIRTH PLAN	97
PREPARING YOUR BODY FOR BIRTHING	100
OPTIMAL FOETAL POSITIONING	101
HOW THE UTERUS WORKS	111
GIVING BIRTH	114
THE FIRST STAGE OF LABOUR	116
SIGNS & STAGES OF LABOUR	117
THE SECOND/ACTIVE STAGE OF LABOUR	124
THE THIRD STAGE	130
THE PLACENTA (AFTERBIRTH)	138
THE BABY	142
EXAMINATION OF THE NEW-BORN	146
NEW-BORN COMMUNICATION	148

CONTENTS

STEM CELLS 153

AFTER THE BIRTH 156

WHEN COMPLICATIONS HAPPEN 159

MEDICAL ASSISTANCE 164

CAESAREAN SECTION 171

PREGNANCY LOSS 181

STILL BIRTH 188

BECOMING A PARENT DURING THE
                COVID 19 PANDEMIC 190

ACKNOWLEDGEMENTS 203

BIBLIOGRAPHY 208

PREPARING FOR CONCEPTION

When most of us arrive in the world, our conception may have been unplanned, accidental, or planned, but often without any conscious preparation for ensuring the maximum opportunity for the unborn child's health at birth, and in the future. The parents' health and well-being are important for the developing embryo or foetus to have the best chance of healthy development. Ideally, you would prepare for pregnancy at least six months beforehand.

It is wise to consult your general practitioner (GP) for a full pre-pregnancy health check as there may be a history of medical conditions relevant to your ability to conceive, and/or carry a pregnancy. It could also include a blood test to screen for your iron level, hepatitis B, chlamydia, syphilis and human immunodeficiency virus (HIV). A healthy, fit body will help to give you stamina for pregnancy, birth, and the subsequent caring of your baby.

It may take longer to get pregnant if you are obese or overweight, so exercise and a healthy, balanced diet are important. Even moderate amounts of alcohol can reduce your chances of conceiving. This applies to men and women - drinking excessive amounts of alcohol can affect sperm count. Smoking reduces your chances of conception, increases your risk of miscarriage during pregnancy, and can harm your baby when breastfeeding.

Check with your GP or pharmacist for the safety, during pregnancy, of any medication you are currently taking; or any new medication or antibiotics, as sometimes you may not be aware you are pregnant in the very early days or weeks. Some over-the-counter medicines can affect fertility and the developing baby, so always check with your health professionals, including getting advice about vitamins and dosages suitable for pregnancy. You should also ask about recreational drugs, such as cannabis, cocaine, and anabolic steroids, which can be harmful to a developing baby.

To reduce the risk of miscarriage, wait three months after stopping the contraceptive pill before trying to conceive. Take folic acid and B vitamins for the first twelve weeks to reduce the risk of neural tube defects, such as spina bifida - maybe sooner if there is a family history. These can be obtained at any pharmacy or supermarket, but it is best to consult your GP or pharmacist.

Consult your medical practitioner if you are on medication for coeliac disease, diabetes, obesity, or epilepsy, or if there is a family history of any conditions that you suspect might be relevant. If in doubt - seek advice.

If a woman contracts rubella (German measles) in pregnancy, especially during early pregnancy, it can cause serious heart, brain, hearing, and sight defects in the unborn baby. This is called congenital rubella syndrome (CRS). If you are unsure of your immunity to rubella, ask your GP to check your immunity status three months before you conceive, and if you are given a vaccination avoid pregnancy for a month afterwards.

A cervical smear test is also advisable before trying to conceive, so early signs of cancer or infection can be treated.

If your work involves exposure to X-rays, pesticides, or anything that might affect your fertility you should ask your GP for advice.

You may need your GP to refer you to a genetic counsellor if there is a history - in either yours, or your partner's family - of medical conditions such as cystic fibrosis, diabetes, or any other known genetic condition.

Make sure you have been treated for any infections caused by sexually transmitted diseases before planning to conceive, as some of these infections can be passed to your baby during pregnancy.

If you can, try to avoid any stressful situations in your life, as stress can affect the hormonal regulation of the menstrual cycle as well as your blood pressure. Seek advice from your GP if you are feeling low or stressed.

If you are having trouble conceiving and wonder if you or your partner might be infertile, your GP can ask for some tests to be arranged. Your doctor will suggest suitable treatment. This could mean:

a) a course of medication to stimulate the ovaries to produce eggs
b) sperm/egg donation
c) intrauterine insemination (IUI)
d) in vitro fertilisation (IVF)
e) adoption or surrogacy could be considered.

Arrange a dental check-up and make sure any dental problems are treated before becoming pregnant.

Resources:

Planning your pregnancy - NHS

www.nhs.uk/conditions/pregnancy-and baby/planning-pregnancy/

A useful site with advice on, healthy eating, foods to avoid, drinking alcohol while pregnant, exercise, vitamins and supplements, stopping smoking, your baby's movements, sex during pregnancy, fertility self-assessment, mental health problems, and how pregnancy affects asthma.

EMMA'S DIARY: PREPARING FOR PREGNANCY GUIDE/PLANNING TO GET PREGNANT/ EMMA'S DIARY

www.emmasdiary.co.uk/getting-pregnant/fertility/preparing-for-pregnancy

A good website all about preparation, pregnancy, birth, and everything related to your baby and more.

THE VOCABULARY OF PREGNANCY AND LABOUR

We may use familiar or private words for the parts of our body. Once pregnancy is confirmed a new set of words will emerge which can be overwhelming and confusing. As the professionals are medically trained they will communicate with each other in medical terms.

Medical terms are not necessarily understood by laypersons, and some words and phrases can be alarming. It is this mystique that adds to the anxiety, tension, and fear of childbirth. It will help you to have translations of the medical terms used, especially during labour and birthing. You can still use your own words and phrases between yourself and your birth companion.

When your pregnancy is confirmed (the word 'diagnosed' immediately has a medical meaning) you will learn your EDD. This is your 'estimated date of delivery' or 'expected date of delivery', with emphasis on the word 'estimated', because there is no exact time for your baby to be born.

A full-term baby can be born three weeks before, or after your EDD. This is the case whether your EDD has been arrived at by ultrasonic scan, or by working it out from the first day of your last menstrual period.

When asked 'when is your baby due?' it is best to be a bit vague about the date, saying, 'sometime in January or February' or whatever month is the closest to the date you have been given. This might avoid the other common remark, 'haven't you had your baby yet?'

The word 'delivery' will be heard frequently by the mother and her partner. To give 'birth' is to give the mother power over her own body, and should replace the word delivery as used by the medical professionals; delivery is a word we associate with a letter or parcel. Delivery also suggests that others, and not the mother are involved with the birth of this baby.

'Birthing' may be a word you prefer to use to describe the period when you and your baby work together with your body to bring your baby into the world. *Women* give birth, and they may feel patronised to be referred to as 'mum' or 'girl'. Ask to be called by your name, the name you prefer to be called by. Professionals are getting better at understanding the importance of showing respect, and the need for consideration of a woman's sensitivity.

As the baby develops, the woman will be examined by a midwife or doctor, by palpating (feeling) the uterus (womb), and expressions such as 'height of the fundus' will be heard. The fundus is the top of the womb and a good place from which to measure the growth of the baby in the womb, as it gradually moves upwards as the pregnancy progresses.

Never be too polite, or shy, to ask questions if you hear words that you don't understand. It is *your* body and *your* baby that is being discussed. Most professionals explain their actions, believing that the expectant parents are entitled to have informed choice in all the observations and procedures involved during pregnancy and the birth process.

LABOUR

The word 'labour' suggests hard work, and in some ways it is, but hard work has its rewards and does not have to be painful. However, labour is the word you will most likely hear from those attending the birth.

The second stage of labour will be referred to as the 'pushing' stage; an alternative word to use is 'easing' the baby out. Easing better describes the expulsive tightening's of the womb which will happen when you are completely relaxed and in the optimal position for labour, without any effort on your part.

MEDICAL TERMS FOR UNBORN BABY POSITIONS

- **OA** - Occipitoanterior - A baby with its head down and it's back between the mother's hip and umbilicus.

- **LOA** - Left occiput anterior - A baby with its head down on the mother's left side, with its back to the front of the mother's abdomen.
- **ROA** - Right occiput anterior - A baby on the mother's right side, with its head down and it's back to the front of the mother's abdomen.
- **OP** - Occipitoposterior - A baby with its head down and it's back to the mother's back.
- **LOP** - Left occiput posterior - A baby with its head down and it's back to the left side of the mother's back.
- **ROP** - Right occipitoposterior. - A baby with its head down and it's back to the right of its mother's back.
- **OL** - Occipito lateral. - A baby with its head down with its back to the side of its mother's abdomen.
- **OL-A** - Occipito lateral - anterior
- **LOL-A** - Left occipito lateral - anterior
- **ROL** - Right occipito lateral
- **RO-P** - Right occipito lateral - posterior
- **Spines** - Ischial spines. Protuberances on either side of the pelvis forming the lower edge of the cavity. Used to assess the descent of the foetus.
- **ARM** - Artificial rupture of the membranes.
- **SRM** - Spontaneous rupture of the membranes.
- **Left Lateral** - Lying on her side position assumed by the mother when in bed that is neither helpful nor hindering to the baby and uterus.
- **Foetus** - This spelling is deliberate. 'Foetus' is the original Latin.

- **'G' Spot** - Nerve plexus at the junction of bladder and urethra. Corresponds to the male prostate gland.
- **Rhombus of Michaelis** - Kite-shaped area at the base of the spine that includes the lower lumber vertebrae plus the sacrum and coccyx.
- **Folding** - The movement of the baby's skull during birth, where bones overlap at the sutures (sutures that separate the bones of the skull).
- **Moulding** - Alteration of the baby's skull bones to reduce its skull diameter.
- **VE** - Vaginal examination

By kind permission of Jean Sutton, author of Let Birth be Born Again.

THE ROLE OF THE PROFESSIONALS

THE MIDWIFE

Midwives deliver most of the babies in the UK, either in a hospital or at home.

It is not generally understood that a woman does not need to consult a medical practitioner, either to have her pregnancy confirmed, for antenatal care and advice, for the birth of her baby, or for postnatal care and advice for mother and baby, while still in hospital and when at home.

The midwife has statutory duties which extend from conception to postnatal care. The midwife is also a member of the obstetric team. The British midwife is legally licensed as a practitioner of normal obstetrics in their own right. Midwifery training is available to men and women, but the majority of midwives are women.

The postnatal duties of the midwife are, that they must be in attendance for not less than ten days, and not more than twenty-eight days, after the birth of the baby. They can use their clinical discretion as to the frequency of their visits, but they must leave an emergency telephone number for contact because midwifery is a twenty-four-hour service.

Midwives can be qualified nurses, a Registered General Nurse (RGN), who have undertaken an extra eighteen months to two years of special training to become Registered Midwives (RM).

Registration is also possible by diploma or degree, and by what is known as a Direct Entry, by completing a three-year or longer training. Midwives can also take other post-registration courses in specialities such as ultrasound scanning, counselling, and specialised neonatal care.

The regulating body for nurses, midwives, and health visitors is The Nursing and Midwifery Council (NMC), which holds the registers of nurses and midwives.

The Royal College of Midwives is a trade union and professional organisation run by midwives for midwives. It provides professional leadership, education, influence, and representation for and on behalf of midwives.

Until 1902, when an Act of Parliament gave midwives sanction to practice, it was the custom for women to be assisted with the birth, and care of their new babies, by laywomen called 'handy-women'.

The word 'midwife' is derived from the Anglo-Saxon words 'mid' = together with, and 'wif' = a woman.

The midwife is trained to recognise the difference between what is normal, and situations where medical or obstetric involvement is necessary. She can refer her client to a GP if there is a medical issue, or to an obstetrician if the pregnancy is outside the normal range.

In general, most women consult their GP in the first instance, and then during their pregnancy and afterwards, their care can be shared between the GP and midwife. In some areas of the UK, all normal births take place in midwife-led units where there are no resident doctors, but the midwives can transfer mothers and babies to medical care if necessary; so you have options to consider.

If the birth is to take place in a hospital, the woman will be referred to a hospital consultant. Unless there are medical or obstetric problems it is unlikely that she will need to see the consultant (specialist), and at her hospital visits, she will be seen by the other doctors in the team. If required she will have total consultant care.

The midwife has special training in the care of the neonate, which is a baby from birth to twenty-eight days old. Their statutory duties are to visit the mother and baby at home on a regular basis, to carry out postnatal checks, and to help and to advise on the mothers and baby's health.

Community midwives usually carry out the home visits but some midwives work in both hospital and homes. They will help with breastfeeding or formula feeding, and establish a close professional relationship with the family to ensure a smooth transition and adjustment to the arrival of the new member.

Ten days after the birth, the midwife will use their clinical judgement to decide whether they need to continue to visit, for up to twenty-eight days, or whether they can transfer care to the health visitor.

In the United Kingdom, maternity care is provided by a team of healthcare professionals, during pregnancy and for some time afterwards.

Childbirth is a natural process and not a medical condition. Too much intervention cascades into more interruptions to the natural processes.

Women were always cared for, at the time of birth, and helped with the care of the newborn baby by other women. Times have changed, and today men are also involved in childbirth and childcare. *At all times, remember that the baby is yours.* Any examinations carried out on your baby - anywhere - must be done in your presence, with your permission, and with an explanation of the reasons for the examination and the expected outcome is called 'informed consent'.

If your rights are not respected in this way, then it is no less than an assault on you and/or your baby.

GENERAL MEDICAL PRACTITIONER (GP)

GPs may have a special interest in one area of their practice, such as obstetrics.

Your GP will inform the midwife who is attached to their surgery or health centre of your pregnancy if they do not already know, and the midwife will refer you to the hospital of your choice - unless you have opted for a home birth. When your baby is born, your GP will be informed of the birth and you will need to register your baby at the medical practice. Your GP may do a home visit, or the midwife will inform him of your progress.

Six weeks after the birth, your GP will carry out your postnatal medical check-up. When your baby is about two months old, your GP will offer you a vaccination programme for your baby.

The British Medical Association (BMA) is the professional association for doctors in the UK.

AN OBSTETRICIAN

An obstetrician is a doctor who has taken further training in the management of gynaecology, pregnancy and childbirth. During your labour, if you give birth in a hospital, you may be seen by any of the medical obstetric team. The consultant usually only attends if there is a complication.

The Royal College of Obstetricians and Gynaecologists (RCOG) is the professional body of obstetricians and gynaecologists. Obstetricians and Gynaecologists are qualified doctors who have undertaken extra training and are qualified to specialise in women's health.

PAEDIATRICIAN

In the maternity unit, the paediatrician is known as the 'baby doctor'. They are available in the labour ward should a problem be anticipated. They check any baby born by caesarean section, or by complicated birth and multiple births. They will also visit any baby the midwife has concerns about.

THE ANAESTHETIST

An anaesthetist only attends a woman in labour if she

requires an epidural, instrument delivery, or caesarean section. Anaesthetists receive up to five years of postgraduate training, depending on their previous experience and training.

THE HEALTH VISITOR

Health visitors are part of the Primary Healthcare team and are usually attached to a particular GP's practice or surgery. Health visitors are qualified nurses who have had one academic year's training in community healthcare. Some health visitors have also completed midwifery training.

Their role is to promote the health of individual families and the public at large. They will follow on from the midwife's visits, will see you and your baby in the 'Baby Clinics', and may even overlap with the midwife, if the midwife decides to continue your care up to twenty-eight days.

They will also be involved with your baby until it is five years old, and are sometimes involved with school children.

HEALTH CARE ASSISTANTS

If you have your baby in the hospital, you will encounter 'healthcare assistants'. Their role is to support the midwives with routine tasks, giving midwives more time for their professional care of the mothers and babies. Healthcare assistants receive
training appropriate to the particular area where they are working. On a maternity ward, this can sometimes include advising on baby care and breastfeeding.

QUALIFIED MIDWIVES

A midwife has acquired the requisite qualifications to be registered and/or legally licensed to practise midwifery. They must be able to give the necessary supervision, care, and advice to women during pregnancy, labour, and the postpartum period.

They can conduct deliveries on their own responsibility, and care for the newborn for up to twenty-eight days. This care includes preventative measures, the detection of abnormal conditions in mother or child, the procurement of medical assistance when required, or the execution of emergency measures in the absence of medical help. The work should include antenatal education and preparation for parenthood, and extends to certain areas of gynaecology, family planning, and childcare.

SAME-SEX PARENTING

Children need to be brought up in an atmosphere of love and care from both parents, and research seems to show that it is irrelevant whether the parents are mother and father, mother and mother, or father and father. Stability and love are the key factors in supporting all aspects of a child's upbringing and happiness.

Very often, couples in same-sex relationships have a desire to have a baby that they can bring up together to complete their family. Adoption is always an option, but they would likely wish for children who has a blood relationship with at least one of them. The answer to that is egg donation for men and sperm donation for women. A woman must provide the egg and a man the sperm, so finding donors must be considered carefully.

Children may ask questions as they grow up, as they do in all circumstances, but as long as they are spoken to openly, and with love and understanding, it should not affect their future relationships with their friends and family.

Although the practicalities of bringing up children are similar to mixed-sex parenting, there are many more considerations and discussions to be faced when embarking on the emotional, and legal aspects of acquiring donor eggs or sperm.

All the health aspects noted in the chapter 'Preparing for Conception' is equally important as for mother/father preparations, although even more counselling, researching, finding the right donor/s, and the legal considerations are necessary and cannot be taken lightly.

For father-father parenting, a surrogate mother needs to be found, and that requires all the legal advice and help, with contracts etc. to be dealt with.

For mother-mother parenting, then it's the sperm donor who needs to be carefully considered, and during her pregnancy and the birth, the partner carrying the baby needs all the care described in this book.

The process may be daunting, but surely worth it when you hold your newborn in your arms. The birth mother can be supported in every way, as described in this book, for the best chance of a safe pregnancy and birth in the best interests of the mother, the baby, and both new parents.

RESOURCES:

OUTCOMES FOR CHILDREN WITH LESBIAN OR GAY PARENTS. A REVIEW OF STUDIES:

www.ncbi.nlm.nih.gov/pubmed/12361102
by N Anderssen - 2002 - Cited by 278 - Related articles

Scand J Psychol. 2002 Sep; 43(4):335-51

A review of studies from 1978 to 2000. Anderssen N (1), Amlie C, Erling AY

Donor Conception Network: Same-Sex Couples

www.dcnetwork.org/same-sex-couples

Alternative Family Law: Legal Paternity after Sperm Donation

www.alternativefamilylaw.co.uk/children/legal-paternity-sperm-donation

'Some women feel uncomfortable with not knowing who the sperm donor is.'

SINGLE PARENTS

You may find yourself becoming a single parent because of a sad loss, broken relationship, by accident, or by choice, and the same practical challenges are present in all cases. There will be things you will need to find out to give yourself the best options to choose from. You are not alone, as statistically there are 1.9 million single parents in the UK.

It will be so much harder if you have lost or broken up with a much-loved partner with whom you may have shared all your excitement, anticipation, and plans for the future. Your heart will be breaking at the thought of going through the experience alone, and you will need all the support and love you can get from family and friends.

If you are a pregnant teenager, don't hesitate to see your GP, midwife, teacher, or trusted friend if you find yourself unable to share your news with your parents or guardians. You may get a lot of support, even if you think otherwise, and although it's hard to take the first step it is better than the loneliness of carrying a secret. Your partner may be very supportive, which is a great help and advantage, and then you must both decide who to share your news with.

It is important for your well-being, and that of the foetus, that you have a medical check-up and professional advice to decide on your options. There is plenty of help and support out there and you will be surprised where you will find it, so embrace it all, and don't be afraid.

There is much to be considered whatever your circumstances. Most important is good antenatal care to ensure the well-being of you, and your future son or daughter - unless there is more than one!

If you are working, there are many options to consider regarding when to return to work, and childcare to arrange, if and when you do so. You have more to think through as a single parent, so finding out what is available as soon as possible, will put your mind at rest. Make enquiries about the rights that are available to single parents, such as entitlement to free dental care and prescriptions, until your baby is one year old.

Help with childcare from parents, family or friends is usually the best arrangement, and most of the time they will love caring for their grandchildren if it is a possibility for them. Not everyone has convenient and willing family members, so there are other, albeit expensive, childcare providers available. Check them out carefully, and be sure that they are licensed with all the legal requirements in place. Visit a few to get a feel for them, examine the facilities, and study factors such as hygiene, staff ratios, qualifications, and how the staff interact with the babies and children in their care. It is hard to be parted from your baby, but as long as you have looked into all the pros and cons you can relax (or at least try to).

Remember - it works well for most parents.

RESOURCES:

HEALTH AND PARENTING: THE TRUTH ABOUT SINGLE-PARENT PREGNANCY

www.health-and-parenting.com/truth-single-parent-pregnancy/

BOUNTY: SINGLE PARENTS

www.bounty.com/family/family-dynamics/single-parents

BABYCENTRE UK: YOUR RIGHTS AND BENEFITS

www.babycentre.co.uk/a562850/your-rights-and-benefits

SURROGACY

A surrogate mother is a woman who has agreed to carry a child through pregnancy and give it up at birth, by pre-arranged agreement, to a couple or single mother who is unable to conceive naturally.

Surrogacy can help childless couples, or same-sex would-be fathers to have the joy of parenthood that they would otherwise have been denied.

Surrogacy is not something to be taken lightly, and there are many bridges to cross on the journey. It is so important to make every effort to ensure everything is legally binding and amicable, as the subsequent child's future needs and happiness are paramount.

Surrogacy can bring immense joy to would-be parents who may have longed for a child for many years. It takes an exceptional person to be a surrogate mother, one who is willing to hand over the baby, nurtured in her womb for nine months, to the new parents. To give such a gift is a wonderful thing to do.

It is hoped that the advice in this book will help the surrogate mother have a good birth and a happy outcome for all concerned.

Under present UK law, the mother who carries the child is the legal parent, and the intended parent must apply to adopt a child born via surrogacy. The intended parent must also be genetically related, either by egg or sperm donation.

RESOURCES:

HAVING A CHILD FOR SOMEONE ELSE (SURROGACY)

https://www.mygov.scot/surrogacy/

SURROGACY UK

www.surrogacyuk.org/

Surrogacy UK, the leading UK not-for-profit surrogacy organisation.

COTS: CHILDLESSNESS OVERCOME THROUGH SURROGACY

www.surrogacy.org.uk/

A leading UK surrogacy support group.

MISCONCEPTIONS OF THE BIRTH PROCESS

Our understanding of the process of giving birth is greatly influenced by the stories passed on by parents, friends, books, films, and television programmes.

Usually, for the sake of dramatisation and sensationalism, birthing is depicted as painful, and there is much screaming, rushing about, noise, and the woman being urged to 'push, push, push!'

If she is in hospital, the woman is usually portrayed lying flat on her back, with all the lights blazing, and everyone is happy when the baby cries loudly. There is an atmosphere of panic with negative anticipation.

Even documentaries, when one would expect to see the reality of birth, one rarely sees a truly gentle and natural birth as nature intended. This would not be entertaining enough, and sadly, leaves young women and their partners with a totally wrong understanding of the way birth ought to be.

Expectant mothers are taught to look forward to pain by friends, family, and health professionals because that has been their experience. People seem to enjoy the attention they receive by relating their negative experiences of birth, sometimes they may even 'embroider' the facts. By the time these stories have been passed around, like 'Chinese whispers', they become more and more dramatic and distorted.

Children who grow up hearing these accounts are conditioned to accept childbirth as painful.

The Bible is quoted to 'prove' that women can expect to give birth in pain as The Curse of Eve (Genesis 3:6). However, modern-day versions of the Bible challenge the many translations with different meanings, placing doubt on the statement, 'with pain you will give birth.' It is more likely to refer to Eve's sorrow and feelings of guilt over her sin in the Garden of Eden, than to the act of childbirth.

Historically, women in labour were attended by other, older women, and birth was conducted in a quiet secluded environment without intervention.

Later, when doctors took over birth, it became fashionable to be attended by a male doctor with women taking to their beds, lying modestly covered, and on their backs, which is not conducive to normal birth.

This added to the tension, fear, and pain, so pain relief was introduced, causing birth to be perceived as a medical condition, requiring hospitalisation, and intervention, rather than a natural function of the woman's body.

Dr Grantly Dick-Read, one of the pioneers of natural childbirth, described how the way giving birth is perceived, from the conditioning we receive in childhood, and all this inappropriate portrayal of this wondrous event, as the 'fear, tension, pain' syndrome.

In other words, pain is caused by tension; tension by fear and 'tense woman means tense cervix.'

He practised the management of normal pregnancy and uncomplicated labour in the belief that intense pain is unnatural and advocated 'natural childbirth' by preparing the mothers with relaxation, exercises, and dispensing with thoughts of painful labour.

Frédérick Leboyer was another 'natural childbirth' obstetrician, and he encouraged a quiet, peaceful and dark environment for birth.

He also introduced immersing the newborn in a bath of deep, warm water immediately after birth to relieve the baby's tension. The warm water, simulating the moist warmth of the womb, helped the baby to experience a gentle introduction to the world.

RESOURCES:

CHILDBIRTH WITHOUT FEAR BY DR GRANTLY DICK-READ - CALM HYPNOBIRTHING

www.calmhypnobirthing.com/childbirth-without-fear-by-dr-grantly-dick-read/

21 Feb 2013 - *Childbirth Without Fear* by Dr Grantly Dick-Read, published by Pinter & Martin Classics, pages 18-19, 2005.

FRÉDÉRICK LEBOYER - WIKIPEDIA

https://en.wikipedia.org/wiki/Frédérick_Leboyer

Frédérick Leboyer (November 1, 1918 - May 25, 2017) was a French obstetrician and autor. He is best known his 1974 book, Birth Without Violence, which popularised gentle birthing techniques, in particular, the practice of immersing newborn infants in a small tub of warm water as a 'Leboyer bath'.

There are many midwives dedicated to the belief that, given the right conditions and support, in most instances, a woman can give birth naturally, and pain-free.

Learning deep relaxation with the help of a birth companion during pregnancy, and enabling an optimal position of the foetus in the uterus by adopting an upright or supported squatting position, provides the best possible chance of natural birth; just as nature intended and which the female body is designed for. Pain is not considered normal in some developing cultures; they cannot afford hospitals and doctors so learn to depend on their bodies to perform the act of birth naturally.

Why should birthing muscles hurt while we are using them when other muscles don't? Other muscles don't hurt when we are using them because they are used voluntarily; they have a different structure to the uterine muscles. Voluntary muscles ache and can be painful if we perform exercises and activities we are not accustomed to, but they do not ache while being used. The pain can be experienced hours after they are over-exercised.

The muscles of the uterus are specially designed for giving birth. They are unique to the womb (uterus). They are involuntary and work on their own accord when triggered by the birth hormones. These birth hormones can be inhibited by the release of the hormone adrenalin, which is produced by fear and tension; abdominal muscles can be affected by tension and fear - all leading to painful labour. Relaxation, and the use of hypnosis, can remove the fear and pain syndrome, allowing the uterine and abdominal muscles to work in harmony with the birthing process.

Childbirth is a normal human function that works without intervention, but too often, intervention is seen as the norm. Intervention interrupts the natural process, and should only be considered where there a genuine medical need.

WISE NUTRITION

Eating wisely in pregnancy, and before conception, is very important to remain healthy and to provide the nutrition your unborn baby needs.

So many new reports and changing advice on the media can be confusing, but a well-balanced diet will help to keep you feeling well and healthy in preparation for the energy you will need not only for your labour but also for feeding and caring for your newborn afterwards.

There are many good sites on the internet that give safe information about the nutrition needed for pregnancy. While you don't need to eat for two, you will feel hungrier. Foods that are nutritious and satisfying are important, and eating three healthy meals a day, starting with breakfast, generally believed to be the most important meal of the day, will provide the nourishment you need.

You should eat a variety of foods: protein, fresh fruit, and vegetables, carbohydrates, dairy foods for calcium, and small amounts of fats, and sugar. Extra vitamins and minerals are essential, as you may not get all you need from your food; therefore, you should take supplements specifically for pregnancy to ensure all your needs are met.

Folic acid is well recognised as an essential supplement to take during pregnancy and, if possible, pre-conception. It is important because folic acid is involved with the development of the brain and spinal cord, and taking a supplement can prevent birth defects, such as spina bifida and hydrocephalus. Your pharmacist can provide you with a suitable dose for pregnancy.

Some raw and uncooked foods should be avoided because of the risk of food poisoning, and meat and fish must be cooked all the way through. Fish, especially oily fish, should be limited because they are now believed to contain pollutants. Unpasteurised cheese should be avoided in pregnancy, and there is a danger of raw eggs containing salmonella, except for eggs produced for the UK under the 'British Lion' Code of Practice.

These eggs come from hens that have been vaccinated against salmonella, and have the 'Red Lion' Quality logo stamped on their shell; these can be eaten raw or partially cooked. Other eggs are best avoided. Be aware that mayonnaise, mousse, and soufflés may contain raw eggs.

Good food hygiene must be always observed, such as hand washing, and cleaning surfaces where food is prepared. Keep raw and cooked foods apart to avoid cross-contamination and, for the same reason, use separate knives and chopping boards for raw and cooked foods.

This is only a brief guide to wise nutrition; more detailed information can be found on the Internet.

RESOURCES:

HAVE A HEALTHY DIET IN PREGNANCY - **NHS** - **NHS** CHOICES https://www.nhs.uk/conditions/pregnancy-and-baby/

WHY DO I NEED FOLIC ACID IN PREGNANCY? - NHS

https://www.nhs.uk/common-health-questions/pregnancy/why-do-i-need-folic-acid-in-pregnancy/

MORNING SICKNESS

It is well-known that sickness and nausea can occur during pregnancy, especially in the early stages. Although commonly called 'morning sickness' it can occur at any time of the day or night and is probably caused by the change of hormones taking place at this time.

Together with tiredness, sickness and nausea are often one of the first signs of pregnancy, although it usually disappears by the twelfth to the twentieth week.

There is little in the way of treatment for this condition, other than to take small meals often, eating a dry biscuit with a drink before getting up in the morning, wearing pressure point wristbands (sometimes used for travel sickness), and eating carbohydrates seems to be more helpful than consuming other foodstuffs, such as fatty foods. In some cases, your doctor may prescribe a short course of an anti-emetic that is safe in pregnancy, but it is best to avoid any medication if at all possible. If the sickness persists (hyperemesis gravidarum) there is a risk of dehydration meaning medical help may be required, or hospitalisation in extreme cases. Thankfully, this is a rare condition and usually soon resolves itself.

RESOURCES:

NHS: VOMITING AND MORNING SICKNESS IN PREGNANCY

www.nhs.uk/conditions/pregnancy-and-baby/morning-sickness-nausea

Coping Strategies for Nausea and Vomiting in Pregnancy

https://www.pregnancysicknesssupport.org.uk/get-help/

Tips on how to cope with pregnancy sickness and hyperemesis gravidarum

Nine morning sickness remedies – Photo Gallery | BabyCenter

https://www.babycenter.com/morning-sickness

Simple, effective remedies that can provide relief from nausea during pregnancy.

EXERCISE

Keeping fit in pregnancy is important. Your body needs to be in good shape, as labour is a physically demanding time.

Walking and swimming are excellent exercises at this time, but if you go to a gym, or have a personal trainer, make sure that they are trained to give you advice for safe exercise during pregnancy. The hormone 'relaxin' makes the ligaments of the pelvis more relaxed and flexible, allowing movement of the pelvic bones during the birth, so care must be taken to avoid strenuous exercise at this time to avoid injury. Some women take yoga or Pilates classes, but contact sport ought to be avoided.

RESOURCES:

NATIONAL CHILDBIRTH TRUST: EXERCISE DURING PREGNANCY: WHAT TO KNOW

www.nct.org.uk/pregnancy/exercise-during-pregnancy

Pelvic floor and stomach exercises in pregnancy. It's not unusual to be worried about the changes to your body that will come from being pregnant.

PSYCHOLOGY

ANTENATAL DEPRESSION (MOTHER)

Becoming pregnant is not always a welcome experience. There are many social, financial, mental, and other health issues that could mean the pregnancy is a cause for concern, and anxiety, especially if it is unplanned. Yet even a planned, and eagerly awaited pregnancy, can give rise to worries, and lead to antenatal depression. If you have a history of depression or have experienced depression with a previous pregnancy, you will recognise the signs and symptoms, which may or may not appear again.

There doesn't even need to be a reason for you to feel down and unhappy when you know you should be making happy plans for the new life within you; it can appear out of nowhere and be difficult to understand and accept.

The huge changes taking place in your body, the rush of hormones brought about by the rapidly developing new life, sometimes causing nausea, sickness, tiredness, and anxiety about all the bodily and lifestyle changes that lay ahead, can provide some explanation. You may have anxieties about the reaction of your partner, and how will he perceive you now, and as the pregnancy progresses: a kind of grief at the loss of the life you have now.

Amidst all the happiness that normally accompanies the news of a pregnancy, there may be lurking uncertainties. All this can lead to depression.

Whether it is called antenatal or postnatal depression (it is still depression, whatever you want to call it), and it needs recognition and treatment.

There are many sources of help for this illness, and you should not be shy or afraid to seek help, firstly from your GP or midwife, who will be familiar with how you are feeling and who will know how to find support, and/or treatment, to make you feel better.

Understanding your antenatal depression or unhappiness will make you aware of the possibility of it happening again postnatally, allowing your obstetric team to keep an eye on you in case you need help after your baby is born.

Talking therapies, counselling, and/or safe medication may be required, and your GP can make a referral for the appropriate treatment for you.

The first and most important step is recognition, and seeking help can enable you to go on to a happy outcome when your baby is born.

RESOURCES:

NHS UK: MENTAL HEALTH HELPLINES

www.nhs.uk/conditions/stress-anxiety-depression/mental-health-helplines/

DEPRESSION ALLIANCE

www.depressionalliance.org

Charity for sufferers of depression. Has a network of self-help groups.

PRENATAL OR ANTENATAL DEPRESSION - PANDAS FOUNDATION UK

https://pandasfoundation.org.uk/what-is-pnd/pre-natal-depression/

At any one time during pregnancy one in every ten women will be depressed and around one in every thirty will be depressed in pregnancy.

ANTENATAL DEPRESSION (FATHER)

It is generally understood that women can suffer antenatal and postnatal depression, but it is not so commonly known that men too can suffer from depression around the time of their partner's pregnancy, and also after the baby's birth. Depression during the pregnancy can continue into the postnatal period and beyond, which is why it is so vital that it is recognised early and treated.

In many ways, men are more vulnerable because they are not being seen and assessed by professionals like their pregnant partner is, who will be seen regularly in clinics, at home, and in hospital, by midwives and doctors, so there are fewer opportunities for the signs to be picked up. All the attention is on the mother-to-be, her health, and that of her growing foetus. This could leave her partner wondering where he fits in with all of this, and feel left out.

Changes in lifestyle and anxieties about the future, such as their relationship, financial concerns, and social changes, plus the responsibilities and anxieties about the health of his partner and baby, all might contribute towards a father's uncertainties.

He will be aware of the media's portrayal of pregnancy and birth, the well-meaning 'advice' of friends and family, and there are times like this when 'a little knowledge is a dangerous thing'. Don't listen to scary stories (people like to dramatise their experiences). Attending good antenatal classes with his partner should help, and sharing his feelings with his partner and GP is also good as well as giving him a chance to get information about the help that is available.

The long term effects and benefits of early diagnoses cannot be exaggerated, and successful treatment is important for good mental health, as well as his life with his partner and their new family, way into the future.

Sometimes friends and family may notice a difference in his behaviour or social habits, and they can be a good support if it's possible to talk to them.

Help is available, so don't be afraid to seek it and avail yourself of it. Please see the links below for sources of help and understanding.

RESOURCES:

ANTENATAL & POSTNATAL DEPRESSION IN MEN | RAISING CHILDREN NETWORK https://raisingchildren.net.au/grown-ups/looking-after-yourself/depression-before-and-after-birth/antenatal-postnatal-depression-men

An Australian website that deals with antenatal depression in men – useful and supportive. If you're a man with symptoms of antenatal depression or postnatal depression (PND), don't ignore them – seek help.

Depression symptoms among men when their partners are pregnant

www.sciencedaily.com/releases/2017/02/170215121044.htm

Elevated depression symptoms for men during a partner's pregnancy were associated with perceived stress and fair to poor health.

HOW THE UNBORN BABY RESPONDS TO STIMULI

Mother and baby bonding begins before birth. Bonding after birth began months before birth, while in the womb, through a communication system established earlier in pregnancy. Dr Stirmann studied the sleeping patterns of newborns. He went on to study the sleeping patterns of the foetus in the womb, discovering how this synchronised with the mother's sleeping pattern, and emotional state.

The foetus seems to be in touch with the mother telepathically, reacting to her emotions, responding to her pain, distress, and the production of her anxiety-activating hormones.

The foetus also responds to the mother when she is relaxed and happy by becoming quiet and relaxed. Many studies have been carried out to prove that there is strong communication between mother and foetus, and birth is a continuation of this. The father too is an important part of this baby bonding, which begins while the foetus is still in the womb. Research has shown that how a man feels about his wife or partner, and their unborn child is one of the most important factors towards the success of a pregnancy. The father's feelings and emotions were disregarded in the past; he is at a disadvantage by not being physically attached to the foetus, as the mother is.

Dr Thomas Verney's studies show that a child can hear its father's voice from the uterus, and researchers have evidence that hearing that voice makes a big emotional impact. In studies, where a man talked to his child in the womb by using soothing words, the newborn was able to pick out his father's voice in a room, even in the first hour or two of life. More than pick it out, the baby responds to it emotionally. For instance, if the baby is crying, and hears his father saying something calming, it will stop; that familiar, soothing sound tells the baby it is safe.

You will become aware of your baby's movements from around the sixteenth or eighteenth week of pregnancy. You will find yourself communicating with your baby by speaking, thinking lovingly, and by putting a hand on your abdomen, stroking and patting it. Your baby will be aware of this and be comforted. This communication becomes even more intense as the pregnancy progresses, and the reassuring messages from you help your baby to feel secure and thrive.

As well as being able to sense your feelings and your love, your baby is sending messages to you, responding to the flow of messages he receives from you by making little movements or kicks. It has been well documented, in hundreds of studies, that unborn babies kick when they are uncomfortable, scared, anxious, or confused. They will also give kicks in response to your communications.

In rural areas of Africa, mothers who carry their babies on their backs are somehow able to tell when their baby needs to eliminate from its bowels or bladder. She senses this need in time to swing the baby off her back, and hold the child away from herself, allowing it to eliminate its waste. If an African woman is soiled by her child of more than seven days old she is considered to be a bad mother. (Dr Thomas Verney)

Studies have also shown that the unborn child can hear from the twenty-fourth week of pregnancy, and after birth, the sounds he has been listening to are familiar but louder. The most familiar, and the most audible, are the sounds of the mother's heartbeat and the rumblings of her digestive and circulatory systems.

All this activity prepares the baby to interact with its parents in the time immediately following birth and its life ahead. The mother's activity level, and emotional state, interlock with the unborn baby's characteristic cycles, as she adjusts to the rhythms of the new life within her; the foetus, in turn, is already experiencing the tempo of her life and through her, that of its father and other family members.

RESOURCES:

THE SECRET LIFE OF THE UNBORN CHILD BY DR THOMAS VERNY, JOHN KELLY

https://www.penguinrandomhouse.com/books/183668/the-secret-life-of-the-unborn-child-by-thomas-verny-md-with-john-kelly/9780440505655/

'HOW YOU CAN PREPARE YOUR BABY FOR A HAPPY, HEALTHY LIFE' A FASCINATING BOOK TO READ.

Study: Pregnant Mother's Touch Elicits Greatest Response From Baby

www.time.com/3930036/mothers-touch-pregnancy-belly

5 Ways A Child Connects With Mother While Being In The Womb

https://blog.parentlane.com/5-ways-a-child-connects-with-mother-while-being-in-the-womb-9491ba866978

22/11/2016 Though initially it might just be a one-way communication, as the baby grows, it can grow to be a fun two-way communication between the mother and the baby. By around 20 weeks, babies start feeling their mother's touch. And when you start feeling your baby move in your womb, touching your baby can be a way to connect with your baby even better.

LOW-RISK PREGNANCY/ HIGH-RISK PREGNANCY

Until recently, all women were encouraged to give birth in a hospital irrespective of whether their pregnancy was considered high or low risk, as the hospital was considered the safest place for all births.

A low-risk pregnancy is one where the mother is fit and healthy with no known medical problems, and it's considered high-risk when a mother might have an obstetric or medical history that could adversely affect the health and well-being of mother and baby.

In the UK, a low-risk pregnancy would mean the birth could take place at home, in a hospital, or a midwifery-led birthing centre, with no need to see a doctor for the whole of the pregnancy and the birth being attended by a midwife alone.

If the pregnancy is diagnosed as high-risk, the mother would be under consultant care and be advised to give birth in a hospital where there are nearby facilities for any medical or obstetric complication that may arise.

At any time during the forty weeks gestation of the pregnancy, the situation can change in both cases and low-risk could become high-risk, and high-risk become low-risk, which is why regular, vigilant antenatal check-ups are necessary throughout this period.

RESOURCES:

WHAT IS THE DIFFERENCE BETWEEN A LOW-RISK AND HIGH-RISK PREGNANCY

www.birthability.co.uk/what-is-the-difference-between-low-risk-and-high-risk-pregnancy/

Low-Risk women can give birth at home, in a midwife-led unit or an obstetric led unit without any prior consultation, and you will be accepted based on your Low-Risk status and can use water if you decide to at any point.

LOW RISK PREGNANCY | **NICE**

www.nice.org.uk/search?pa=1&ps=15&q=low%20risk%20pregnancy

LOW RISK PREGNANCY - **NHS EVIDENCE**

www.evidence.nhs.uk/search?q=low%20risk%20pregnancy

Alternative versus standard packages of antenatal care for low-risk pregnancy Source: Cochrane Database of Systematic Reviews - 16 July 2015 programmes with reduced visits for low-risk women with standard care.

TYPES OF BIRTH

VERTEX – HEAD-FIRST

This is the most favourable position for birth. There are variations of the head-first presentation, as the baby can lie in different positions, but most are with the baby's back facing the mother's abdomen.

Fewer than 10 per cent of babies are born back to back (with their back towards their mother's back), which can result in a long and difficult labour.

Adopting the optimal foetal position, as described in this book, can avoid the baby getting into this position before labour begins.

RESOURCES:

BABY POSITIONS IN WOMB: WHAT THEY MEAN - HEALTHLINE

www.healthline.com/health/pregnancy/baby-positions-in-womb

The baby is facing head down, but their face is positioned toward your abdomen instead of your back. This is typically called the occiput-posterior (OP) position.

BABYCENTRE UK - GETTING YOUR BABY INTO POSITION FOR BIRTH

www.babycentre.co.uk/a544493/getting-your-baby-into-position-for-birth

POSTERIOR|SPINNING BABIES

www.spinningbabies.com/learn-more/baby-positions/posterior

BREECH PRESENTATION - FEET, FOOT OR BUTTOCKS FIRST.

In the past, babies presenting in the breech position were delivered vaginally by doctors and midwives, but it is now considered obstetrically safer to deliver these babies by caesarean section.

The obstetrician may try to turn the baby at about thirty-six weeks gestation by an ECV (external cephalic version). This will be successful in about fifty per cent of cases and the birth will take place with the baby in the head-down position.

If the ECV procedure fails, and the baby does not turn spontaneously, a caesarean section will be advised. The baby will be fine, but may have its legs in the 'frog' position for a few days until they straighten out; this causes no ill effects.

RESOURCES:

WHAT HAPPENS IF YOUR BABY IS BREECH? - NHS

www.nhs.uk/conditions/pregnancy-and-baby

Babies often twist and turn during pregnancy, but most will have moved into the head-down (also known as head-first) position by the time labour begins. However, that doesn't always happen, and a baby may be: bottom first or feet first (breech position).

BREECH BIRTH - BABYCENTRE UK

www.babycentre.co.uk/a158/breech-birth

Find out what it means if your baby is in a breech position.

PRECIPITOUS LABOUR

A birth is described as precipitous labour if a baby is born less than two hours after the first twinge of contractions; this is extremely rapid, and in some cases, it is even quicker. This can happen in about two per cent of all women, and the mother may be unaware that contractions are occurring, or may think she is having Braxton Hicks contractions. These are tightening's of the womb from late pregnancy onwards, sometimes described as 'practice' contractions.

The disadvantages of a precipitous birth are that the mother and baby are vulnerable because there is not enough warning for any preparation to take place or to go to a safe environment, and these births can happen when the mother is alone, in a car, car parks, trains, buses, and even aeroplanes.

It may be reassuring to know that a precipitous birth is usually without complications. All that is needed is calmness, to keep the baby warm by holding it close to your body, and to send for help as soon as possible. There is no need to cut the cord as is commonly supposed, but to keep the placenta (afterbirth) at the same level as the baby, if possible.

Resources:

Precipitous Labor: Everything You Need to Know | Parents

https://www.parents.com/pregnancy/giving-birth/labour-and-delivery/precipitous-labour-everything-you-need-to-know/

While most labours stretch several long hours, some women experience a "precipitous labour" that only lasts two or three hours. Fast labour seems great at first glance (fewer contractions and less pain!)...

BIRTH OPTIONS

NATURAL CHILDBIRTH

Natural childbirth means birth without medical intervention, or intervention of any kind, and can occur in a hospital or the home.

You need the right environment, education, and the freedom to adopt the optimal position during labour/birthing to allow the baby to emerge easily. A quiet, calm environment is essential, with the mother-to-be adopting whichever position she finds most conducive for her comfort. Thus allowing the foetus to adopt a favourable position in the womb for an easy entry into the world, and following the mother's instincts without the restraints of intrusive examinations, and the restrictions of being confined to bed.

The safety and well-being of mother and baby can be observed by the midwife or attending professional who will, respecting the mother's privacy and dignity considering the stage of labour she has reached, document the vital signs of mother and baby between contractions with the minimum of disturbance.

Natural birth means a birth that empowers you to be in control of your own body, by giving you the confidence to trust that the female body is physiologically equipped to bring forth a new life with the minimum of stress.

The achievement of a natural birth begins with pregnancy, learning about the changes happening to the body during pregnancy, the process of birth, removing any pre-conceived negative beliefs, and learning to relax in preparation for the birth of the baby.

Your feelings and wishes must be communicated to the professionals involved in your care and their co-operation gained. It is most important to have a suitable birth partner, who may be a husband or partner or a special friend or relative: someone who is committed to, and fully understands the importance of their commitment, to give support during the pregnancy and birthing process.

By learning how the body changes in pregnancy to support and protect the growing foetus and the mechanisms of the birthing process, which is designed to soften and stretch to allow the baby to ease out gently, you will learn to trust your body and will develop a partnership with your baby, both working in harmony to bring your baby into the world. It only needs those people close to you at this time to respect your wishes and to support you in achieving your aim.

COMPLICATIONS

Sometimes, although no one's fault - least of all the expectant mother - a helping hand is needed. Only the professional carers present at the time can identify reasons why the natural process of birth is not taking place as expected, and hopefully, a good rapport will have developed so that you, and your birth companion, will trust the professionals in their judgement and take their advice.

However, a clear explanation should be given to you and your birth companion, and help given only when the professionals have obtained permission.

Remember, the outcome aimed for is a healthy mother and a healthy baby, and all interventions are not necessarily going to prevent natural childbirth; in some cases it may be necessary, to allow the birthing to go on to a successful natural, relaxed birth. Learning relaxation techniques during pregnancy, and/or hypnosis will help during any procedures that may be required. So long as an explanation is given at all times, and it is an informed choice, it is best to take good advice when it is given.

If a caesarean section becomes necessary, you should not feel guilty, or that it is your fault, in any way. There are many reasons why help may be needed, some of which are caused by the shape of the pelvis, the size or condition of the baby, and the health of the mother. Remember, the priority is a healthy mother and, a healthy baby.

In all circumstances, knowledge and understanding of how the body is working and how the baby is involved with this, together with all that has been learnt about relaxation, will help.

You and your partner should be encouraged to enjoy your baby just as you would if everything had gone according to plan. If you have needed help with one baby it does not mean that you will automatically need help with subsequent babies. Every pregnancy and every birth is different.

Learning relaxation techniques during pregnancy, and/or hypnosis will help during any procedures that may be required. So long as an explanation is given at all times and it is an informed choice, it is best to take good advice when it is given.

HOME BIRTH/NATURAL BIRTH

Any woman with a low-risk pregnancy may wish to have a home birth, but bear in mind that during any pregnancy conditions can change, and a low-risk pregnancy can become high-risk and high-risk can become low-risk, depending on many circumstances; every person and every pregnancy is different. Of course, the mother's health and the progress of the pregnancy will be monitored throughout and any changes observed.

After decades of women being strongly advised that hospital was the safest place of birth, following several studies there has been a change in opinion, and now those women fulfilling the low-risk category are fully supported by NHS trusts' policies. The National Institute for Health and Care Excellence (NICE) recommend home birth for women with low-risk pregnancy because there is less risk of intervention and infections. NICE recommend that all women should be supported and be free to choose their birth settings. There is more risk of baby and mother contracting infections in the hospital.

It is usual for two midwives to attend to women for a home birth. However, at present, there is a shortage of midwives in the UK. Rarely, but it has been known to happen, two midwives are not available, so a hospital birth or birth centre becomes an alternative option. Thankfully this is rare.

You have four options for the place of birth for your baby:

> Hospital, under the care of an obstetric consultant (although most babies are delivered by midwives, and it is more likely you will not need to see a consultant).
>
> A midwifery-led unit in a hospital setting close to the hospital facilities.
>
> In a midwifery-led unit or birth centre.
>
> In your own home, with midwives in attendance.

To some extent, the area where you live will affect your options for the location of birth, as available facilities can vary in different areas.

Midwives are in charge of their units and birth centres, but they always have access to medical help if it is required. They can summon medical help at a home birth if it's needed, just as they can in a hospital.

Midwives are legally required to stay with a woman in labour even if she refuses medical advice or hospital care, but a doctor can refuse to attend if his advice has been rejected. It is illegal for an unqualified person to attend a woman in labour and to deliver a baby, except in an emergency, but it is not illegal for a mother to choose to give birth without assistance.

If your midwives have concerns over your health or that of your baby at any time during your labour, they can arrange for you to be transferred to a hospital.

ADVANTAGES OF HOME BIRTH

When your contractions have started and you are in established labour, you do not have to be disturbed by preparing for and travelling to the hospital. If you have other children, they can stay at home, in bed if it's night-time, and experience the wonderful meeting with the new baby when they wake up.

In your own home, you are in familiar surroundings so can relax better. After the birth, you and your partner do not have to separate and can enjoy your baby together.

You have a better chance of having a midwife that you got to know during your pregnancy, and there is less likelihood of intervention, forceps, etc. than with a birth in hospital.

If you wish to have a water birth you can hire one for the occasion, which can be set up in your home. Your midwives can give you pain relief should you need it, such as 'gas and air', medication by injection, massage, or anything that you find helpful
and relaxing, but you cannot be offered an epidural analgesia at home. You can employ a doula or family member to give back-up to your partner.

RESOURCES:

AM I ALLOWED? AMAZON.CO.UK: BEECH, BEVERLEY LAWRENCE

www.amazon.co.uk/Am-Allowed-Beverley-Lawrence-Beech/dp/1874413150

Beverley Beech is our long time legendary campaigner for women's rights in pregnancy and birth, skilled international orator, researcher and writer based on almost 40 years' experience in advising parents about their rights. Am I Allowed? is a must for any pregnant woman who wants to exercise informed consent and be more in control of her pregnancy and labour. It gives you the information to make YOUR informed decision.

ASSOCIATION FOR IMPROVEMENTS IN THE MATERNITY SERVICES

www.aims.org.uk

AIMS is a volunteer-run charity campaigning on maternity issues, supporting home birth, and providing birth information and support via a helpline and a website.

NICE RECOMMENDS HOME BIRTHS FOR SOME MUMS - NHS

www.nhs.uk/news/pregnancy-and-child/nice-recommends-home-births-for-some-mums/

Home births have dominated the UK media today, following the publication of guidance by the National

Institute for Health and Care Excellence (NICE) on the care of healthy women and their babies during childbirth. The main talking point was the recommendation that women thought to have a low risk of pregnancy complications would be better served by giving birth at home or a midwife-led unit, rather than at a hospital.

UNASSISTED BIRTH

It is not illegal for a woman to decide to birth to her baby without midwifery or medical assistance, this is called *free birth*. While supporting a woman's right to make this choice, midwifery, and medical organisations, will advise mothers of the risks involved for both mother and baby. However, it is a legal, informed choice in the UK.

The registrar holds the legal responsibility for recording all births, but it is legally the father's responsibility to report the birth to the registrar. In reality, this is often carried out by the midwife in attendance at the birth.

It is confusing, as this is new since I did my training. The exception is if the woman is considered to have mental health issues. A midwife cannot refuse to attend a woman in labour or antenatal care, as a doctor can. MG

RESOURCES:

FREEBIRTH, UNASSISTED CHILDBIRTH AND UNASSISTED PREGNANCY | **AIMS** www.aims.org.uk/information/item/freebirth

What are free-birth and unassisted childbirth? There is no specific definition of free-birth, but broadly speaking, a woman free-births when she intentionally gives birth to her baby without a midwife or doctor present. Some women prefer to use the term 'unassisted childbirth' or UC to describe this.

UNATTENDED OR UNASSISTED BIRTH IN THE UK | ASSOCIATION OF RADICAL MIDWIVES

www.midwifery.org.uk/articles/unattended-or-unassisted-birth-in-the-uk/

AIMS advises any woman who is told that "if we have a shortage of midwives at the time of your labour you will have to come into hospital" to write a short letter back stating that they have no intention of coming into hospital and they expect a midwife to attend when called.

UNASSISTED CHILDBIRTH STATEMENT - DOULA UK

www.doula.org.uk/statement-on-unassisted-birth-with-doulas-present

HOSPITAL BIRTH

You can choose to give birth in the hospital, and you may have a choice of hospitals depending on the area where you live and the availability. Most women chose this option but you can change your mind during your pregnancy depending on the status of your pregnancy.

You can still aim for a natural birth if you choose the hospital option.

In hospitals in the UK, most babies are delivered by midwives, but doctors are available and you have the facilities of the hospital should you need help. Your obstetric team will answer your questions on what is offered. Very often a tour can be arranged so you can look around, see the birthing rooms, and get an idea of what to expect when you are admitted.

Most hospitals have birthing pool facilities, as well as other birth aids, such as birth balls and comfortable chairs. There might be a limited number of birthing pools in the unit so it could be first come, first served.

You may still choose to have a natural birth in the hospital with or without hypnosis, a birth doula, or another birth companion. All your choices and desires should be written on your birth plan and noted on your records, which will be carried by you.

ADVANTAGES OF HOSPITAL BIRTH

- You have immediate access to an obstetrician if your birth becomes complicated and an anaesthetist if you choose to have an epidural anaesthetic.

- If your baby needs a little help or a lot of help, there are paediatricians and neonatologists on hand and, should it become necessary, your baby will be close to the special care baby unit, with incubators and specially trained staff to care for your baby.

- If all is well with the mother and baby, you may go home within a few hours or, depending on the time of day, be admitted to a postnatal ward until you are ready to be discharged.

DISADVANTAGES OF HOSPITAL BIRTH

Intervention is more likely in hospital, possibly leading to breaking the waters surrounding the baby, epidural anaesthesia, forceps or Ventouse assistance.

There is no reassurance of seeing a midwife who is familiar to you from your antenatal clinics, so you could have a midwife who is a stranger to you. However, it does not take long to develop a rapport with your midwife.

There is a risk of you or your baby developing a hospital infection during your time there, which is why it is advisable to go home as soon as you are both ready.

ADVANTAGES OF HYPNOSIS IN CHILD BIRTH

It is our birth right to come into the world in a calm, stress-free atmosphere.

Hypnosis promotes relaxation, allowing the mother to follow her inborn instincts. Relaxation allows her body to work as nature intended, which eliminates the fears leading to tension and pain during childbirth.

Birthing is a joyful and safe experience in a natural, relaxed atmosphere. It allows the body to work in harmony, without resisting the natural contractions, leading to the thinning and opening of the womb, and the birth of the baby. The involvement of the birthing partner is crucial.

Hypnosis reduces the exhaustion resulting from a long period of 'pushing', as when the mother is sufficiently relaxed the 'pushing' phase of the birthing happens without strenuous effort. The womb will gently push the baby into the world naturally, as being relaxed allows the structures to stretch slowly and without incurring damage. The mother is less tired and stressed, and can enjoy and bond with her baby.

Because stress and fatigue can be experienced without this kind of support, postnatal depression may also be reduced. The need for medical interventions, the use of drugs, and other artificial aids are reduced and frequently eliminated, having no after-effects for mother or baby from the use of drugs for pain relief or an epidural.

Choose a programme that combines hypnosis with full antenatal information for you, and your chosen birth companion, to prepare you mentally and physically for the birth, thus enabling you to fully visualise everything that is happening to your body.

Some medical conditions contra-indicate the use of hypnosis, and some people are not suitable as candidates for personal reasons.

RESOURCES:

RESEARCH ON THE USE OF HYPNOTHERAPY IN PREGNANCY AND CHILDBIRTH

Evidence-Based Research Studies - Hypnobirthing Utah
www.hypnobirthingutah.com/evidence-based-research-studies-supporting-the-use-of-hypnosis-for-childbirth-preparation/

Evidence-Based Research Studies Supporting the use of Hypnosis for Childbirth Preparation February 28, 2011 Hypnosis: practical applications and theoretical considerations in normal labour.

HYPNOSIS IN CHILDBIRTH RESEARCH - HYPNOBIRTHING

www.hypnobirthing.co.uk/hypnosis-in-childbirth-research

Links to scientific research articles about hypnosis and hypnotherapy in labour and childbirth.

WATER BIRTH

Michel Odent is an obstetrician who, in 1977, worked in a hospital in Pithiviers in France. He installed a pool to help his patients with pain relief and rest when the labour was long and difficult. It has since become popular worldwide. Many maternity hospitals are now providing birthing pools in their birthing rooms and maternity centres.

Relaxing in warm water is very comforting during labour and babies can be born in the pool, or you may wish to get out for the actual birth, it is your choice depending on your feelings. It is perfectly safe for your baby to be born into the water, for while the cord is still attached, the baby is receiving oxygen from the placenta.

It is important that your midwife understands the safety aspects of water birthing, and has received training in this practice: being aware of temperature, hygiene, and safe pain relief. It is not advisable to use narcotic pain relief, but 'gas and air' (nitrous oxide) and hypnosis are safe.

If you are planning on a home birth, it is possible to hire a birthing pool but for a hospital birth, you may be limited to the availability of the pool as they may not have one in every birthing room.

RESOURCES:

BIRTH UNDER WATER - MICHEL ODENT - ACTIVE BIRTH POOLS

www.activebirthpools.com/birth-water-michel-odent-2/

Blog: 12.10.2016. Michel Odent's ground-breaking report "Birth Under Water" that was published in The Lancet in December 1983 is widely regarded as the seminal moment in time when the use of water for labour and birth entered our consciousness.

WATER BIRTHS EXPLAINED - MUMSNET

www.mumsnet.com/pregnancy/labour-and-birth/water-birth

A water birth is a safe way to have your baby and is increasingly common and popular. As the name suggests, it involves giving birth (or labouring) in water - usually in a specially designed pool. The comforting sensation of warm water can help you relax during labour and even reduce labour pains and the need for pain relief.

THE HISTORY OF WATER BIRTH - ACTIVE BIRTH POOLS

www.activebirthpools.com/history-water-birth
www.activebirthpools.com/category/active-birth-pools-info

IMMERSION IN WATER IN LABOUR AND BIRTH | COCHRANE

www.cochrane.org/CD000111/PREG_immersion-water-labour-and-birth

16 May 2018 - To assess the effects of water immersion (waterbirth) during labour and/or... more about the benefits of water immersion in labour and birth for women... further research is needed particularly for waterbirth and its use in birth...

CASCADE OF INTERVENTION

Intervention in pregnancy means applying medical techniques or artificial hormones to induce labour, or to augment labour if the process slows down. Whatever method is used, and for whatever reason, it interferes with natural birthing.

Some situations may arise during, or at the end of pregnancy when intervention may become necessary. Because there is a risk either to the mother or baby, such as pre-eclampsia in the mother or if the baby is failing to grow in the womb because the placenta is not functioning properly; there are many other examples. In these cases, there is no other option but to intervene and all explanations should be given by the attending professionals.

It has been explained earlier, that the EDD is only an estimate of the day the baby will arrive. If there are concerns for the health of the baby before the EDD and the birth is induced, depending on the number of weeks into the pregnancy, the baby may be born premature and need special care. This situation is unavoidable.

Some establishments have protocols determining the number of weeks over the EDD when inducement of labour will be advised, and it can be a dilemma for the mother-to-be. It is possible if the EDD has been wrongly assessed, for a baby to be born before it has finished its development in the womb, causing it to be preterm unnecessarily.

When the EDD has passed, and there is still no sign of labour starting, there is concern that the baby may be post-mature. When the baby has developed enough to begin life in the outside world, the things that have sustained it in the womb will start to deteriorate. The placenta, which has completed its job, will stop functioning properly.

The fluid surrounding the baby, and the white, creamy vernix caseosa which surrounds the foetus from about week eighteen, will decrease, and the bones of the foetal skull will harden, making it more difficult for the overlap to take place at the moment of birth.

If the onset of labour is thought to be late, the first method that may be suggested is sweeping the cervix. The doctor or midwife will sweep a gloved finger between the cervix and the membrane surrounding the baby, without breaking the membrane. This is supposed to stimulate prostaglandins, the hormones thought to start the process of birth by softening and thinning the cervix. This is painless for some but painful and uncomfortable for others. It is only thought to work if the cervix is 'ripe' and ready to efface and dilate anyway.

Prostaglandins are present in semen, which is why mothers are sometimes encouraged to have intercourse if the baby is 'overdue'.

These are all procedures that can be classed as interventions, but which may also be medically necessary to preserve the health of mother and baby.

Likewise, once labour is in progress, other interventions may be felt necessary to preserve the health of mother and baby, but all too often they become routine because it is convenient for labour to have a time limit.

The cascade of intervention was described by the midwife, Sally Inch, in the early 1980s in her book, *Birthrights: What Every Parent Should Know About Childbirth in Hospitals*. It describes how intervening can lead to more and more intervention, leading to all possible scenarios from instrument birth to caesarean section.

RESOURCES:

BIRTHRIGHTS: WHAT EVERY PARENT SHOULD KNOW... - KIRKUS REVIEWS

www.kirkusreviews.com/book-reviews/sally-inch/birthrights-what-every-parent-should-know-about/

24 Jan 1984 - BIRTHRIGHTS: What Every Parent Should Know About Childbirth in Hospitals by Sally Inch, a childbirth educator in England, has deftly incorporated the English experience into her discussion without losing sight of the American scene. What she displays is a 'cascade of intervention'.

FIRST DO NO HARM: INTERVENTIONS DURING CHILDBIRTH - NCBI - NIH

www.ncbi.nlm.nih.gov/pmc/articles/PMC3647734/

By L Jansen - 2013 - Cited by 25 - Related articles

Although medical and technological advances in maternity care have drastically reduced maternal and infant mortality, these interventions have become commonplace if not routine.

INDUCTION

Induction of labour means intervention during the pregnancy by methods such as rupturing the membranes (breaking the water) or medical procedures to induce uterine contractions, to bring about the birth of the baby

Induction may be advised for post-term pregnancy or for concerns that continuing with the pregnancy would risk the health of the mother or baby. You will need to be admitted to the hospital so the well-being of you and your baby can be monitored throughout the procedure.

The method of induction of labour can be a vaginal pessary containing the hormones necessary to stimulate the onset of contractions, or by intravenous infusion of the hormone oxytocin, which will usually have a quicker action. The method employed is decided on the circumstances of each individual case, but you will be under the care of midwives and obstetric medical staff until the birth of your baby and afterwards.

RESOURCES:

What is Induction of Labour? | Information for the Public

www.bcu.ac.uk/health-sciences/business-and-innovation/partnership-opportunities/ebmbc/centre-staff/jane-denton

What is induction of labour? Labour is a natural process that usually starts on its own. Sometimes labour needs to be started artificially; this is called 'induced labour'.

Induction of Labour - Indications - Risks - Procedure

https://teachmeobgyn.com/labour/delivery/induction-of-labour/

12/05/2018 Induction of labour (IOL) is the process of starting labour artificially. Whilst most women will go into labour spontaneously by week 42 of gestation, roughly 1 in 5 pregnancies will require an induction. As a general rule, IOL is performed when it thought that the baby will be safer delivered than remaining in utero.

Inducing Labour - NHS

www.nhs.uk/conditions/pregnancy-and-baby/induction-labour/

If you're being induced, you'll go into the hospital maternity unit. Contractions can be started by inserting a tablet (pessary) or gel into the vagina. Induction of labour may take a while, particularly if the cervix (the neck of the uterus) needs to be softened with pessaries or gels.

THE CERVICAL SWEEP

This is a common procedure as the first option for induction.

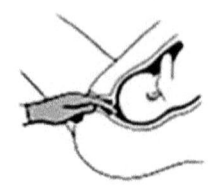

Illustrated by Laura Bagnall, Valdark Illustrations

A 'sweep' or 'stretch and sweep', is a procedure carried out by a midwife or doctor to stimulate the cervix and initiate labour. The lubricated, gloved finger of the professional sweeps between the cervix and the amniotic membrane. The finger is inserted into the opening of the cervix to slightly stretch it, which is believed to stimulate the hormone prostaglandins and induce labour. It has variable levels of success.

RESOURCES:

CERVICAL SWEEP | EVIDENCE SEARCH | NICE

www.evidence.nhs.uk/search?q=CERVICAL%20SWEPw

Does a cervical membrane sweep in a term healthy pregnancy reduce the length of gestation?

Membrane Sweep at 37, 38, 39, 40 Weeks, Success Rate

https://brighterpress.com/women%2Fpregnancy%2Fmembrane-sweep-38-39-weeks-success-rate-risks

14/01/2018 The procedure involves the following steps: An obstetrician will explain what will happen during the procedure, as well as the length of time it... If you experience any discomfort, you will be encouraged to take shallow, relaxed breaths.

BIRTH PARTNER/COMPANION

Research has shown that there are many benefits to the mother and baby if the mother has a supportive birth companion. This can be a person chosen by the woman to be someone she feels comfortable with, and trusts as a reliable committed person to share her birth experience with. It does not necessarily have to be her husband or partner.

The birth companion can support both the woman and her partner, or work as the sole supporter if the partner is absent by choice, or by mutual agreement.

The husband or partner is not always the best person to be around at the time of birthing, not through lack of concern but perhaps because his close relationship with his partner could cause him anxiety. He will need support from elsewhere and be prepared to share in the joy and celebration afterwards. His support will also be needed with the care of the newborn in the future.

The birth partner will have a very special relationship with the woman, and her partner, if present, must also be very comfortable with the birth partner. The pregnant woman should consider very carefully who will be best to offer her comfort, support, and praise throughout the birthing process. Equally, the birth companion must feel comfortable in a situation that is very personal, intimate, and something to be remembered for a lifetime.

The reliability and commitment of the birth

partner are essential, and there must be absolute honesty if they feel, at any time, that this commitment is more than they can give. If there are any second thoughts they should be expressed as soon as possible, while there is still time to find a replacement. This is vital as the birth partner needs to attend every antenatal class with the mother to be, as they both need to learn the techniques required for a natural birth. The birth partner has to be one hundred per cent certain that they want to share in this wonderful event in this special way.

The woman will depend on the birth partner to guide her through the advice shown in this book as she progresses through the birthing process. The birth partner must support the woman to achieve the choices she has made and written on her birth plan and to support her if, for some reason, she is advised that some things on the plan are not possible.

The birth partner must also be prepared to speak up for the woman's needs and wishes, and therefore needs a certain degree of assertiveness. The mother-to-be will need the encouragement and advocacy of her birth partner for the duration of the birthing process. The birth partner will be with the mother-to-be the whole time, as long as it takes, for the all-important techniques that both have learnt.

The midwife will, of course, also be present to give support all of the time, but in an hospital birth, they may have to leave if the shift ends before the baby arrives, so the birth partner is the one constant companion.

If the baby's father is also there, the birth partner can give him a break if he needs to leave to care for other children, make phone calls, or any other business. Also, he can be there for the birth partner to take a short break for essential reasons.

RESOURCES:

CONTINUOUS SUPPORT FOR WOMEN DURING CHILDBIRTH | COCHRANE

www.cochrane.org/CD003766/PREG_continuous-support-women-during-childbirthhttps://www.cochrane.org/CD003766/PREG_continuous-support-women-during-childbirth

Continuous support during labour may improve outcomes for women and infants, including increased spontaneous vaginal birth, shorter duration of labour, and decreased caesarean birth, instrumental vaginal birth, use of any analgesia, use of regional analgesia, low five-minute Apgar score and negative feelings about childbirth experiences. We found no evidence of harms of continuous labour support.

BIRTH PARTNERS - ROYAL COLLEGE OF MIDWIVES - RCM | EVIDENCE

www.rcm.org.uk/media/3887/birth-partners.pdf

Royal College of Midwives - RCM source - 17 April 2020 - Publisher: Royal College of Midwives

Having a trusted birth partner present throughout labour is known to make a significant difference to the safety and well-being of women in childbirth.

ROLE OF THE BIRTH PARTNER DURING THE BIRTH

HOW TO ASK QUESTIONS AND BE POLITELY ASSERTIVE

The role of the birth partner is to give support and advocacy to the woman and her partner (if appropriate) throughout the pregnancy and birthing experience.

The birth partner needs to be aware of, and in harmony with, the woman's needs and wishes, and to be able to make a commitment for the duration of the pregnancy and the birthing process, whenever it occurs and for however long it takes.

The father of the baby may be the birth partner, but there should be no pressure on him to do so, or for him to feel guilty if either parent feels he is not the right person. Everyone has different needs and experiences which can affect them at this time, and which must be respected.

The birth partner will be in a position to make the needs of the woman known to the professionals in attendance, and that may require the need to be assertive at some stage. The nature of the birth process is such that the hormones flowing at that time can cause the woman to be unable to think clearly.

Having to make rational choices or communicate effectively will interrupt the natural release of hormones, and could result in the birthing taking longer than necessary. The woman in labour must be allowed to concentrate on giving birth without outside interference of any kind unless it's medically necessary. She can be assertive in pregnancy, but when giving birth she must be left in peace to follow the dictates of her body.

The birth companion should have had an opportunity to visit the hospital, or other places of birth, in order to be familiar with the surroundings beforehand, and should also have a copy of the birth plan with them as an 'aide memoire'.

During the birthing (assuming it is in hospital) a friendly and co-operative attitude towards the staff, and acknowledging the unique position of the midwife in being able to help with the goals of the birth plan, will help to maintain a relaxed atmosphere. The midwife will be needed as an ally to ensure that the mother's wishes are always observed so that when the couple arrive at the hospital, or if a home birth, they should discuss the birth plans and request her help. Explain to the midwife that the mother wishes her companion to act on her behalf so that she is disturbed as little as possible.

It is important to be aware of the language used when speaking to the staff thus avoiding unrealistic requests, angry tones, or loud demands as these will arouse hostility and not help to maintain a calm, peaceful atmosphere. Being assertive is difficult in unfamiliar surroundings leaving the woman feeling vulnerable and insecure, but the birth partner is there to protect the mother-to-be and she is relying on them to prevent any disturbance and to provide her with the right environment for her baby's birth.

Creating good communication and openness is always better, letting the people doing their job know how the mother-to-be wants things to go. They can only help if they are told, clearly and politely, what they need to know.

Enquiries made at the right time, without interrupting the staff too frequently will ensure their respect, as they too will be anxious to make the experience a memorable event. Every effort to adhere to the birth plan must be made, but the birth partner must listen carefully if reasons to change direction are given, making sure they understand and agree with the explanations.

They must ask questions if they see actions which they are unsure of, or that they might not understand. Their involvement in all stages of the pregnancy, the relaxation exercises and the preparation of the birth plan will give them the confidence of informed choice.

RESOURCES:

TIPS FOR YOUR BIRTH PARTNER - **NHS**

www.nhs.uk/conditions/pregnancy-and-baby/what-your-birth-partner-can-do/

Whoever your birth partner is - the baby's father, a close friend, partner, or a relative - there are many practical things they can do to help you. The most important thing your birth partner can do is just be with you. Talk to your birth partner about the type of birth you'd like and the things you prefer not to do so they can help support your decisions.

BIRTH DOULA

A Doula is a woman who supports families during the period of pregnancy, birth and the postnatal period. She may, or may not have medical qualifications, but could have taken a course of Doula training and is possibly a mother or grandmother herself.

This training is not regulated and there are many different formats, so some research is necessary to be sure you make the right choice. Ideally, in addition to some training or relevant qualification and experience, anyone working with babies and children should have the recognised police checks (the Disclosure and Barring Service currently in 2020), which are very easily obtained by prospective employers, and it is advisable to obtain evidence of this to ensure you employ a suitable person.

Some doulas specialise in supporting mothers and their partners for the birth, which usually includes visits during the pregnancy and in the postnatal period, depending on your individual arrangements. Other doulas work with families in the postnatal period, giving support after the baby is born, helping with breastfeeding, general baby care, and sometimes helping with other children.

The birth doula will stay with you for the duration of your labour, helping and supporting you and your partner. She could be your birth partner if you wish. Doulas are self-employed and usually charge an hourly or fixed rate for a birth booking.

RESOURCES:

WHAT IS A DOULA? | NATIONAL CHILDBIRTH TRUST

www.nct.org.uk/pregnancy/who-will-care-for-you-during-pregnancy/what-doula-your-questions-answered

A good source for information in pregnancy, breastfeeding and all aspects of baby care.

WHAT DOULAS DO - DOULA UK

https://doula.org.uk/what-doulas-do/

Birth doulas provide continuous support, for women and couples, through pregnancy, labour and birth and in the immediate postnatal time.

COULD A DOULA MAKE YOUR BIRTH BETTER? | MOTHER&BABY

www.motherandbaby.co.uk/pregnancy-and-birth/birth/getting-ready-for-birth/doula-hire-could-a-doula-make-your-birth-better

'Doula' is a Greek word for a care-giver. We have no specific medical training and will not give medical advice or instruction during birth. A midwife's job is to focus on the safe delivery of the baby, whereas a doula's job is to support the mother emotionally. There are two types of doulas - birth and postnatal.

"A doula is there to support the mother, meet her needs and provide constant reassuring," says Himalee Rupesinge, Recognised Birth Doula (Doula UK).

PREPARING A BIRTH PLAN

Whether the birth is to be at home or in hospital it helps to have a written plan of your hopes and preferences for how you would like your birthing to happen.

Contact the midwife and ask if you can discuss your plan with them beforehand. A copy can be given to the midwife and one kept in your notes, but it will help if you can discuss your plan with the midwife beforehand if that is possible.

The plan should also be discussed with your midwife, to confirm if they have problems with any aspects of it, then any issues can be resolved before the baby's day of birth.

You may see more than one midwife during your pregnancy. There is not always continuity of care during the antenatal period so more than one midwife may be seen during pregnancy. If the plan is clearly written, it may also help to highlight and prioritise important points, to help the birth attendants comply with your wishes.

Most babies in the UK are helped into the world by midwives who are the practitioners of normal birth, but they are qualified to recognise if help or medical intervention is necessary. At present, The Royal College of Midwives is currently focusing on their *Better Births* initiative so a request for a natural birth should be welcomed. Midwives are also required to comply with evidence-based practice, which means they have to justify their actions concerning the research which has proven it is a safe practice. As well as this, they have to adhere to procedures and protocols laid down by the hospital trusts which employ them. They are also accountable for their actions to the general public via The Nursing and Midwifery Council, which is the regulating body.

When the plan is written, it is good for you to be able to make informed choices, and it is easy to find information by reading, researching on the internet, attending appropriate courses, and reading this book. If the midwife is presented with the evidence supporting your wishes, it puts you in a stronger position, making for a good working relationship between you and your birthing attendants, meaning your birth plan will be welcomed as helpful.

It will help to write the plan in such a way that the midwife can use their professional judgement in certain situations, so long as you have been given an explanation and are reassured that, even if it is not what you had originally hoped for, it is in the best interests of you and your baby. With the best will in the world, there are occasions when an unexpected situation arises but hopefully, with the relaxation techniques, and knowledge learnt at classes, or from this book, and the help and support of your chosen companion, the chances of surprises are greatly reduced.

You and your partner need to gather information from women you know who have had babies, (but do not listen to 'horror' stories), or from antenatal appointments, as well as researching on the internet. You should talk to the person who is going to be your birth companion and make notes as they come to mind, so they can be written up and be referred to later.

You will be given your maternity notes, which contain information about you and your pregnancy, to keep with you, and you may get some ideas from the information therein.

As the birth is planned as a natural birth with the help of relaxation techniques (learnt by you and your companion), you will need to include the birthing positions you wish to adopt as part of your plan, to enable you to give your baby the optimal foetal position for an easier birth. This needs to be made clear on the plan.

An important part of care while birthing is the monitoring of the foetal heart rate at regular intervals. The midwife can do this by using a hand-held device called a 'Sonicaid', or by electronic monitoring which uses straps to hold electrodes in place. If you wish to remain free and mobile, you would be best advised to request a handheld device. Some centres have more choice in foetal heart monitoring to allow you to stay mobile. You may be asked to stay on the bed for about twenty minutes for a read-out from the monitoring machine which, as well as counting the foetal heartbeat, also traces the strength and timing of the tightening of the uterus and the reaction of the foetus to the tightening. This is a useful guide and base to start with, and should not interfere with your wishes to remain mobile after it is completed.

You may wish to use a birthing pool, which many enjoy. You should seek as much information as you can about the pros and cons of this choice, so you are well prepared.

When planning a natural birth it would seem appropriate to follow it with a natural birth of the afterbirth (placenta). This is called the third stage and a natural third stage is called a physiological third stage of labour.

The common alternative to a physiological third stage is the use of a drug called Syntometrine, given by injection into the mother's thigh as the baby is emerging from the birth canal. The action of Syntometrine is to speed up the birth of the placenta by making the uterus squeeze it out in a shorter time than the natural way, and is also believed to reduce blood loss. It could be necessary for this drug to be given at some stage, even if the woman has opted out of the birth plan, but the reason for this will be explained by the midwife and permission sought.

Becoming informed beforehand makes it easier to make good decisions.

There is strong evidence about the cutting of the umbilical cord, which has sustained the foetus during its life in the womb, and of waiting until the cord has stopped pulsating before it is cut, which means the blood flow from the placenta has ceased.

There is also research that favours putting the baby straight onto your chest or abdomen, but of course, this is a personal matter and needs to be on the birth plan. This is the time when your baby looks for their first feed, and your wishes regarding breastfeeding or formula feeding need to be made clear.

If at any time, the unexpected should happen,

then you may wish to make a note of your preferences in your plan, but without hindsight, it may be best to trust your professional attendants to keep you informed and to explain clearly any action which deviates from your birth plan that they consider necessary. Always remember that the safety and welfare of the mother and baby are their first consideration.

If you have any special health needs, the health professionals need to be made aware of them to give the best possible care, but this will have been dealt with at the initial consultation with your doctor, or midwife when the pregnancy was confirmed.

You may be invited to take a tour of the place where you plan to give birth, especially if you are a part of a group or antenatal class. This would be a chance to familiarise yourself with some of the staff and the environment, and allows you the opportunity to ask questions about such things as your birth plan, what birthing equipment is available, birthing pool availability, movement in labour, help with breastfeeding, and many other questions personal to your individual needs.

Never be afraid to ask questions of the midwives or doctors; this is a very special time in your life and knowledge is power. Understanding what is happening makes for a more relaxed and pleasant atmosphere.

The list of wishes that could be put on a birth plan is endless, but if it is too long it could be difficult for the birth attendants to take it all in, as their main objective is care and safety. Nevertheless, you have rights and must not fear being assertive in expressing your wishes, while still maintaining a good relationship with the professionals. This will ensure a happy birthing experience for all concerned.

RESOURCES:

STATEMENT ON RCM'S BETTER BIRTHS INITIATIVE

rhttps://www.rcm.org.uk/media-releases/www.rcm.org.uk/media-eleases/2017/august/statement-on-rcm-s-better-births-initiative/

14/08/2017 The Normal Birth Campaign was focused on birth. The Better Births Initiative encompasses pregnancy, birth and the postnatal period. The Better Births Initiative seeks to improve care for all women, including those with medical and obstetric complications. The focus of the Better Births Initiative is to ensure the best birth for all women. One example of this would be to encourage women in labour to remain mobile.

MAKING A BIRTH PLAN - NHS

https://www.nhs.uk/conditions/pregnancy-and-baby/how-to-make-birth-plan/

Find a birth plan template and learn about making a birth plan, including where to give birth, pain relief options, who to have with you and your feelings.
Where to give birth ·What your birth partner can do ·Pain relief in labour.

WATER BIRTH PROS AND CONS: SHOULD YOU HAVE A WATER BIRTH?

www.goodtoknow.co.uk/family/water-birth-79850

What are the pros of having a water birth? Pain relief. Being in warm water can make it easier to deal with painful contractions. If you want strong pain relief... Enhanced sense of privacy. Once you are in the warmth of the pool you can focus solely on the labour.

Latest recommendations on timing of clamping the umbilical cord | RCM

Quality statement 6: Delayed cord clamping | Intrapartum care

www.nice.org.uk/guidance/qs105/chapter/quality-statement-6-delayed-cord-clamping

10/12/2015 Rationale The benefits of delayed cord clamping include higher haemoglobin concentrations, a decreased risk of iron deficiency and greater vascular stability in babies. If they wish, women can ask healthcare professionals to wait longer to clamp the cord.

Clamping of the Umbilical Cord and Placental Transfusion | RCOG

www.rcog.org.uk/en/guidelines-research-services/guidelines/sip14/

SUGGESTIONS FOR YOUR BIRTH PLAN

.... wishes for a Natural Birth with the help of:

Clinical Hypnosis (optional) and Optimal Foetal Positioning

.... has been practising self-hypnosis (if appropriate) to prepare for the contractions when labour begins. She wishes to avoid all other medication.

.... has attended all childbirth preparation sessions and is helping .... with her (hypnosis).

.... will be .... birth partner and advocate during the birthing process.

The expertise and advice of the midwives in attendance will be respected at all times, and their advice will be followed after an explanation for any deviations from the birth plan.

Requests:

......................, as a birth partner, will be the conduit for communication with ....

A quiet, calm and peaceful environment with subdued light, but bearing safety for midwives' observations in mind.

.... to be disturbed only when if necessary, to allow her to give all her attention to her relaxation and working with her body while giving birth.

Mobility during labour or positions which .... finds most comfortable, including lying on a mattress on the floor in a left lateral position.

Minimal vaginal examinations or other interventions.

Avoid artificial rupture of membranes (breaking water bag) unless medically indicated.

Non-directed pushing (see an article in references) allowing ....to listen to her body.

Allow transitional pause between first and second stage, to give the foetal head time to descend onto the perineum, unless .... naturally feels expulsive contractions and the cervix is believed to be fully dilated.

Natural third stage (birth of placenta), so no Syntometrine unless medically indicated.

...........................would like to cut the umbilical cord, if possible.

Skin-to-skin contact after the birth, for as long as possible, to initiate breastfeeding, leaving as much vernix on the baby as possible.

Private time for ...., ... and baby, with unlimited refreshments and tea or coffee.

Refreshments for all midwives and the obstetric team and a big Thank You!

This is ONLY a guide: you can make changes and add more as you WISH.

PREPARING YOUR BODY FOR BIRTHING

Pregnancy and birth are natural events in a woman's life. You need to be prepared physically and mentally for the act of childbirth. Great physiological changes are imposed on a woman's body during this period. Some effort and work is required - which may be why the word 'labour' is used! Lead a quiet life, with plenty of fresh air, and walking or swimming daily.

One of the pregnancy hormones - relaxin, softens ligaments and supportive tissues, thus reducing the stability of joints throughout the body. This hormone allows the bones of the pelvis to give, allowing more room for the emerging baby. Some form of exercise to strengthen the muscles involved in birthing is a good beginning and should be instructed by a person professionally qualified to ensure the safety of the exercises.

A reputable programme of exercise especially for pregnant women should only be conducted by instructors who are aware of these bodily changes, to avoid dangers to joints, especially of the pelvic girdle and spine.

And a healthy, balanced diet is also an essential part of keeping fit.

OPTIMAL FOETAL POSITIONING

THIS IS A PIONEERING CONCEPT DEVELOPED BY NEW ZEALAND MIDWIFE JEAN SUTTON.

Jean believes it is important to understand the relationship between the mother's pelvis and the head of the foetus and how it affects the birthing process.

Modern lounge furniture which inclines backwards are particularly bad for mothers-to-be in the last weeks of pregnancy.

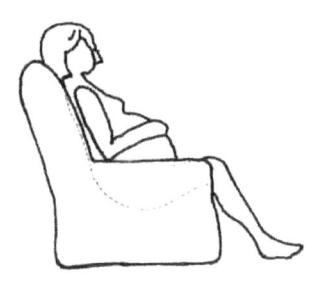

PROPERLY DESIGNED MATERNITY STOOLS

Maintains the lumber lordosis (the curve of the lower spine which occurs in pregnancy), encouraging the baby to take up the optimal foetal position for easier birthing.

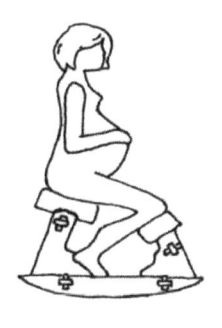

BIRTHING POSITIONS

Good Position For Resting, and During Pregnancy and Labour.

To encourage the foetus back and away from the mother's back, lay on the left side.

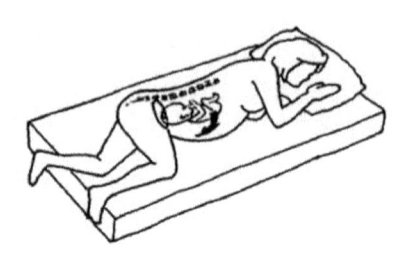

At this time, adopting appropriate positions to help the foetus get into the final ready-to-birth position avoids causing the foetus to take up a position more difficult to obtain an easy birth.

BIRTHING POSITIONS

(a)

Standing

Good Lordosis

Mother upright and forward

Plenty of space between spine and symphysis

Baby supported by mother's abdominals

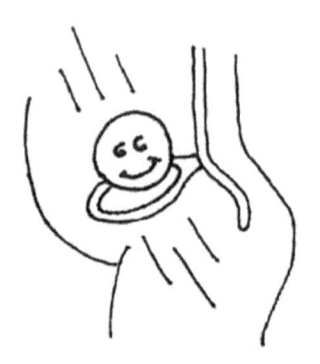

(b)

Sitting

Little or no Lordosis, with baby in O.P. position

Inlet level, preventing baby bringing back forward to allow head under sacrum

MAY ENTER IN LABOUR

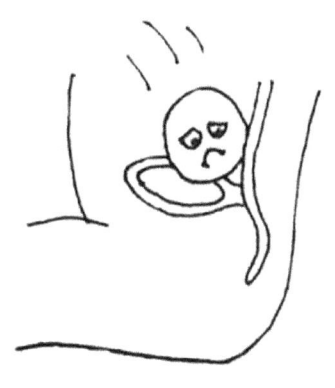

(c)

Squatting - Western women bring spine forward & bottom down, closing the inlet & tightening the pelvis floor.

This is not advisable

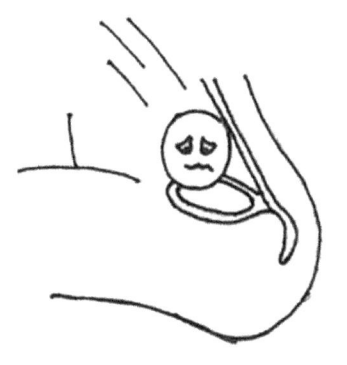

BIRTHING POSITIONS EXPLAINED

(a) This is a good position for the mother to adopt in labour. Lordosis, the inward curvature of the spine which occurs in pregnancy, helps to keep the baby forward and allows space between the spine and the bone at the front of the pelvis, called the symphysis pubis. The baby is supported by the abdominal muscles.

(b) Sitting positions are not good to adopt in labour. Sitting pushes the baby into the OP position (occiput posterior) which means that the baby's back and head are against the mother's back, preventing the baby from bringing its back forwards to allow the head under the sacrum. (The sacrum is the wedge-shaped bone at the end of the spine which moves up to give more room for the baby to be born.)

(c) Western-style squatting is not a good position; bringing the spine forward and the bottom down closes the inlet and tightens the pelvic floor. This is not advisable. Eastern-style squatting is different and is the position adopted by many Eastern cultures for many activities. Their bodies have adapted accordingly, but western cultures have not physically adjusted to this position.

Positions adopted during pregnancy and birthing will help the foetus adopt the optimal position, allowing the maximum space to enable natural progress through the pelvis and birth canal.

By thirty-six to forty weeks into the pregnancy, the baby takes up more room than the fluid surrounding them. It is now that the mother's positions can help the baby get into the best position for an easier birth.

The ideal position for the foetus to take up immediately before birth is the left occiput anterior, with the baby with its head down, lying on the mother's left side and with its back to the front of the mother's abdomen.

FULL-TERM BABY

Baby with its head down on the mother's left side, and

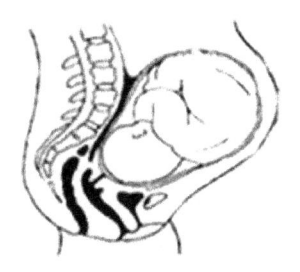

with its back to the front of the mother's abdomen.

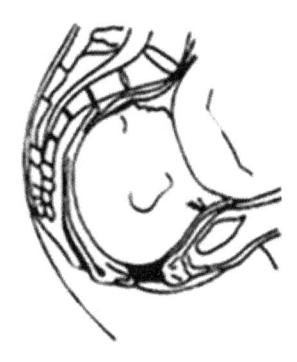

With the uterus low and the cervix pointing in the correct direction, with a little bit of help, the foetus will try to move into the optimal position.

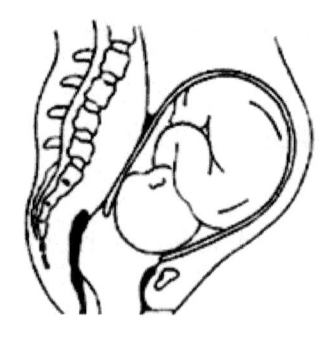

Cervix fully dilated - note position of the posterior lip of cervix. Engagement and rotation complete - note nose is on top of the sacrum

(The sacrum is the triangular bone at the base of the spine that joins to a hip bone on each side and forms part of the pelvis.)

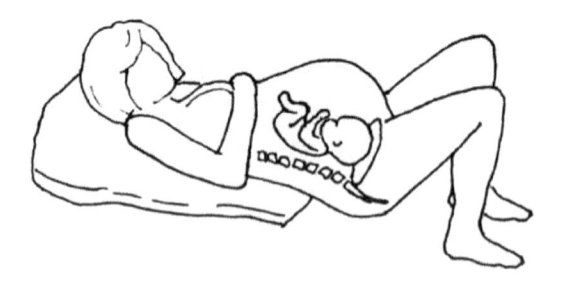

Lying flat on her back is a bad position for a pregnant woman

    The weight of the developing foetus can cause pressure on a large vein called the *inferior vena cava*, slowing down the flow of blood back to her heart. This is a common cause of low blood pressure and results in a feeling of faintness.

The woman lying flat on her back in late pregnancy encourages the foetus to lie with its back to the back of the mother, which is not conducive to a good birthing.

Likewise, modern-day armchairs which incline backwards may be very inviting to relax in and to put one's feet up, but they have the same negative effect on the position of the foetus.

During the last trimester of pregnancy (final three months), it is advisable to spend some time lying on the left side and practising upright and forward-leaning postures.

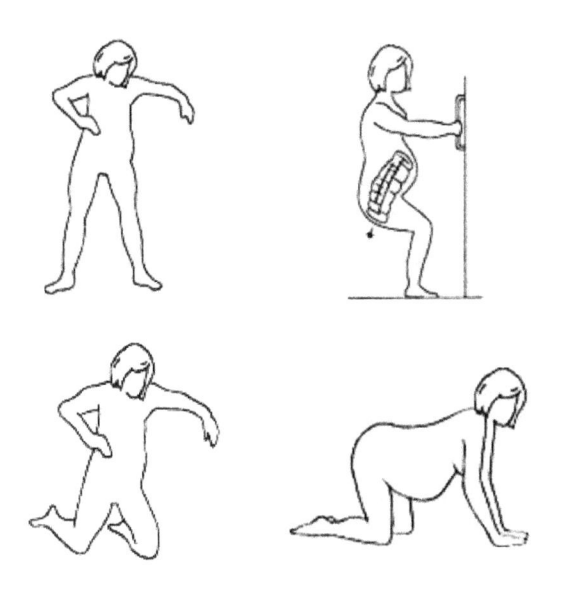

Images sourced from Let Birth be Born Again by Jean Sutton. By kind permission of Jean Sutton

RESOURCES:

MOTHER'S SLEEPING POSITION AND RISK OF STILLBIRTH - NHS

www.nhs.uk/news/pregnancy-and-child/mothers-sleeping-position-and-risk-of-stillbirth/

Widespread media coverage has been given to a study on the risk of stillbirth and the sleeping position of the mother. "Mums-to-be should sleep on their left side", reported The Mirror. The Daily Mail said, that "women who sleep on their right side or back during the late stages of pregnancy could be at higher risk of stillbirth."

A recent study has caused some concern in the media as it showed a link between mothers who slept on their backs during pregnancy and a higher risk of stillbirth, but the studies were not conclusive and require more research.

The study was carried out by researchers from the University of Auckland and the Wellington Medical School in New Zealand. It was published in the **'peer-reviewed'** *British Medical Journal.*

WHAT MOTHERS NEED TO KNOW

- Birth is a co-operative action between mother and baby.

- The baby tries very hard to assume the best position for birth.

- The woman must, if possible, keep her knees lower than her bottom.

- When resting, she should lie on her left side with her legs level with her body.

- Her baby's efforts to turn across her pubis will vary between uncomfortable and painful.

- She can minimise this pain by adopting forward-leaning postures while her baby is moving.

- There is no point in trying to move her baby when it is sleeping. Wait till it awakes.

- When her abdomen sags and her back aches, it is better to wear a girdle than to tuck her tail under. Expect some lordosis (forward curvature of the spine).

- Once her baby is in the best position, the only small lump she will feel is far around between her hip bone and ribs

- A baby in the best position gives good signals to its mother's body, to prepare to let him out easily for both of them. Remaining upright and mobile will aid labour.

- This baby is likely to be born on time and proceed as the books tell us.

- It will come out with a minimum of effort, in as short a time as possible, and arrive peaceful, unstressed and ready to get on with life.

- Chemical pain relief is not likely to be needed, as the mother's body will respond to her baby's signals and she will cope magnificently.

Sourced from Let Birth be Born Again - By kind permission of Jean Sutton

HOW THE UTERUS WORKS

The non-pregnant uterus is a hollow, muscular organ measuring 7.5cm long, 5cm wide and 2.5cm deep. Each wall is 1.25cm thick. It weighs 60g, and at the end of the pregnancy, as a result of the hormones produced, it grows and stretches and weighs 900g and measures 30cm x 23cm x 20cm The cervix or neck of the uterus protrudes into the vagina.

The uterus, or womb, provides a protective and nutritive environment in which the foetus develops and grows. It has a very special arrangement of muscle layers which all have a particular function during labour.

When it is time for the baby to be born, the hormones produced in pregnancy will help the womb to tighten, or contract, rhythmically from the top (fundus) to the bottom part. The top muscles tighten to squeeze the baby down, and the lower muscles help to draw up the cervix and dilate it or open it up, for the baby to come through. At the same time, the cervix is pulled up or effaced, until it becomes thin and dilated. The tightening feels like a strong wave beginning at the top and spreading down to engulf the whole uterus, and then it fades and relaxes. The sensation can be felt in the back and/or the thighs.

The tightening's last for about thirty seconds, every fifteen to twenty minutes, at the beginning of labour, to fifty to sixty seconds, every two to three minutes towards the end. They become stronger and occur at more regular intervals as labour progresses.

The progress of labour is measured by the dilatation of the cervix, which can be assessed by vaginal examination, with the mother's permission. The cervix is fully dilated at 10 cm when there is sometimes a pause before the second stage of labour, which is the 'pushing' stage, and every tightening or contraction becomes expulsive, to push the baby down the birth canal (vagina) to be welcomed into the world.

The uterus is perfectly designed to fulfil its function, and the baby's skull bones are perfectly designed to overlap, to allow the head to come through the birth canal. The ligaments supporting the pelvis soften in pregnancy and move to allow the baby through the birth canal.

There is increasing evidence to suggest that active pushing with contractions when the cervix is fully dilated is unnecessary and that the expulsive contractions will happen naturally allowing a more gentle birth. However, these studies have shown that the second stage of labour will be longer.

The bag or membrane containing the fluid or liquor that the baby lies in may remain intact throughout labour. It does not have to be artificially broken (ruptured) unless there are signs that the baby is in distress, such as when the baby has had its bowels opened. Only the health professional in attendance can advise if this occurs.

It may be suggested to the couple that breaking the membrane containing the foetal fluid surrounding the baby will speed up labour, and this is correct - but it can also increase the strength and intensity of the tightening's. If the woman is relaxed and coping well with labour, there is an advantage in a longer, calmer, more natural birth with an intact membrane, allowing the uterus to gently push the baby out without active pushing.

GIVING BIRTH

New Zealand midwife, Jean Sutton, describes the Rhombus of Michaelis, the area of the spine which moves back up to 2cm, and described to Sheila Kitzinger by Jamaican midwives, as the mother 'opening her back,' giving extra space for the baby to emerge.

Next comes the 'Foetal Ejection Reflex' described by Michel Odent, as the mother moves her body, maybe thrusting her hips forward, for the baby to emerge: the spine lifts, the coccyx moves upwards and her back arches for the baby to emerge. To allow this to happen, the position of the mother is important; she should be preferably supported standing or squatting.

After the birth, the mother needs to stay relaxed to allow the placenta (afterbirth) to come away.

If the baby needs aftercare, in a hospital setting they may need to be placed on a baby trolley, which is usually kept in the birthing room. The baby trolley has an overhead heater to warm the baby up (if necessary) and is equipped to provide the care and attention the baby may need. It is best to allow the midwife to deal with this situation, should it be necessary, knowing the baby is in safe hands, while the completion of the natural birth takes place.

Michel Odent, obstetrician and advocate of natural birth, believes that the first hour after birth is very important, and is the beginning of the mother-newborn interaction. The mother and baby gaze at each other and hormones are released which, as well as playing the part of love and bonding, also help with the expulsion and the commencement of lactation (production of milk in the breasts).

Given the opportunity, in the right circumstances, the baby can find the breast in the first hour after birth, and the sucking action of the baby and the warm, quiet, relaxed environment can aid the expulsion of the placenta and even reduce the amount of bleeding.

THE MUSCLES OF THE WOMB

Outer Longitudinal Muscle Fibres

Middle Muscle Fibres

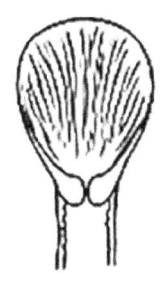

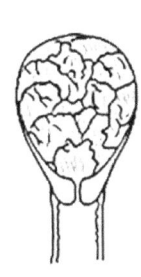

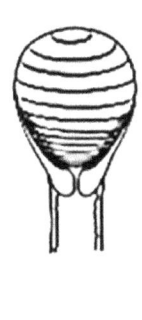

Circular Muscles Fibres - Found in the Lower Part of the Womb

Illustrated by Laura Bagnall, Valdark Illustrations

THE FIRST STAGE OF LABOUR

The first stage of labour is defined as the beginning of regular contractions of the womb until full dilation of the cervix is 10cm dilated.

PATTERN OF CONTRACTION DURING THE FIRST STAGE OF LABOUR (BIRTHING)

The contraction starts at the top of the womb and spread across the fundus. The shaded area shows the contraction getting stronger as it spreads over the womb. The lighter area shows the contraction fading and getting weaker and finally in the resting phase.

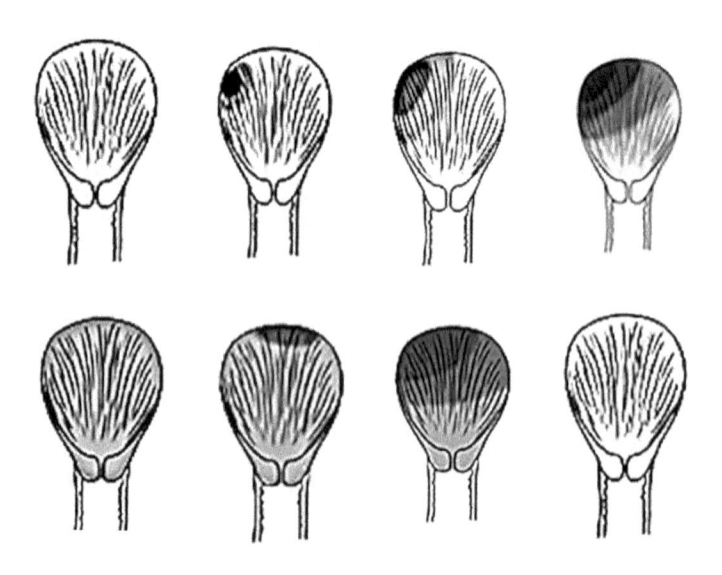

Illustrated by Laura Bagnall, Valdark Illustrations

SIGNS AND STAGES OF LABOUR

'Birth is an involuntary process, and as such cannot be managed.' (Michel Odent; Hawaiian Conference 1995)

SIGNS THAT LABOUR HAS BEGUN

1. Regular contractions or tightening of the uterus.

2. A 'show', which is a small amount of blood occurring when the plug of mucous sealing the cervix comes away taking some blood with it. This is not necessarily a sign of immediately impending labour, although it may be; it can occur three to seven days before labour becomes established. It does, however, mean that changes have started to take place in the cervix. It is wise for the midwife to be informed.

3. Rupture of the membranes, or 'breaking of the waters', experienced by a gush of clear fluid which cannot be controlled (unlike urine) meaning the membrane surrounding the foetus has broken, releasing the amniotic fluid. The midwife should be told immediately as there is a small risk of the umbilical cord being swept down with the fluid.

These events can occur in any order and do not necessarily mean that labour has started, but it is important that the woman be seen and checked by her midwife. Regular contractions becoming stronger and more frequent is a positive sign.

THE STAGES OF LABOUR

Once labour has become established, the majority of women will experience the birthing process as a continuous process that increases in intensity up to the moment of birth. I have divided it into three stages for easier understanding. The timings vary and can be different for each woman, and even different pregnancies.

FIRST STAGE

Vague backache; intermittent cramps similar to menstrual cramps which may extend to the thighs; restlessness or a burst of energy called the 'nesting instinct' can all be early signs of labour.

The backache can continue, with contractions/tightening's radiating from front to back, and gradually progressing to becoming longer and stronger and closer together. When the contractions are regular and it becomes difficult to be distracted, labour can be said to be established: the cervix is becoming soft, effacing and dilating. This stage can last from two to twenty hours, and may be longer for first-time mothers but not always.

Throughout labour, the midwife will be monitoring the progress and well-being of the mother and baby, taking her temperature, pulse and blood pressure at regular intervals. She also needs to listen to the foetal heartbeat every fifteen minutes.

The midwife may want to do a vaginal examination to assess the progress of the dilatation of the cervix, for which she needs the mother's permission and for which the mother needs an explanation. She will monitor the strength and frequency of the contractions, and how they are affecting the foetus and will encourage and support the mother as labour progresses.

ENTONOX (GAS AND AIR)

Entonox is a gas taken by inhalation via a special mouthpiece or mask and is a mixture of 50% Nitrous Oxide gas and 50% Air, which will be offered at any time during labour. It does not affect the baby and is only effective whilst being inhaled.

It is self-administered, and as it induces drowsiness the mouthpiece is released, the air is breathed, and you become fully awake. It is a very useful aid to help throughout labour and does not prevent you from going on to enjoy natural childbirth.

Entonox is used by dentists and paramedics and is commonly called 'laughing gas' because it has a somewhat euphoric effect on the receiver.

PETHIDINE

Pethidine is a drug offered when labour is established, and if the contractions have become uncomfortable

and difficult to manage. It is given by intramuscular injection in the thigh and the effect lasts for about four hours. It can help to give you some respite if labour is long, and it gives you a chance to have a little rest and replenish your energy.

It is best not given too close to the anticipated birth, so you can be awake and alert to take full part in the birth of your baby; as it can affect the baby after birth, causing sleepiness and slow to establish feeding. Nausea can be a side effect.

You are most likely to be asked by your midwife for your permission for her to carry out a vaginal examination for an assessment of your cervical dilatation. Receiving pethidine can still allow you to go on to have the natural birth you have planned.

You are most likely to be asked by your midwife for your permission for her to carry out a vaginal examination for an assessment of your cervical dilatation. Receiving pethidine can still allow you to go on to have the natural birth you have planned.

STAGES OF CERVICAL DILATATION

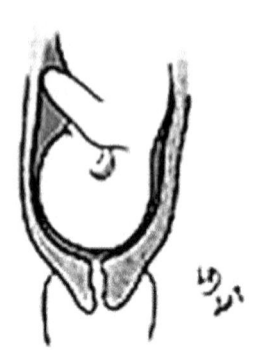

Cervix long, closed and uneffaced

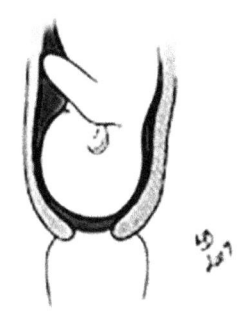

Cervix taken up, some dilatation has occurred

Illustrated by Laura Bagnall, Valdark Illustrations

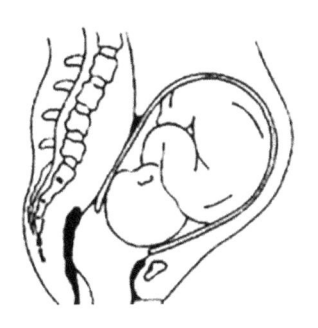

Cervix fully delated at 10 cm

Illustration from Jean Sutton

BIRTHING POSITIONS

GOOD POSITION FOR RESTING DURING PREGNANCY AND DURING LABOUR

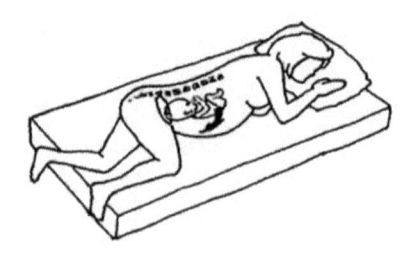

BAD POSITIONS FOR THE MOTHER AND THE BABY DURING LABOUR

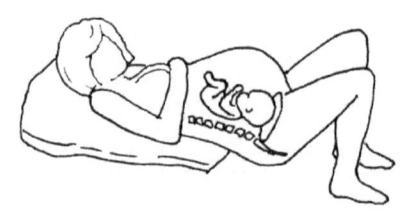

Reclining causes more problems than it solves

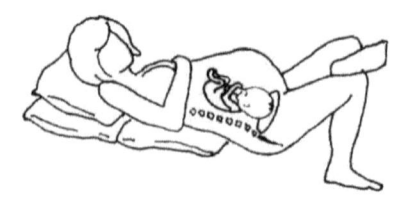

This is a bad position in late pregnancy and labour, as it encourages the baby to lie with its back to the mother's back.

Images Sourced from Let Birth be Born Again by kind permission of Jean Sutton

THE AMAZING RHOMBUS OF MICHAELIS

We are never taught about the rhombus and its crucial role in second-stage labour.

The way out for the baby is head down, facing backwards, so it can follow the pelvic curve. The rhombus is a bit like a jigsaw - the pieces may look the same, but there is only one space they will fit into without using force.

At the beginning of the physiological second stage of labour, this area moves backwards to increase the outlet for the baby from 13 cm to 16 cm. The widest part of the pelvic outlet is 13 cm if the woman is sitting on her coccyx, or lying on her back, thus preventing this movement of these spinal bones.

HOW THE RHOMBUS OF MICHAELIS WORKS

This is the kite-shaped area that includes the three lower lumbar vertebrae and the sacral prominence. As the sacrum is effectively fused, the whole posterior pelvic wall is involved.

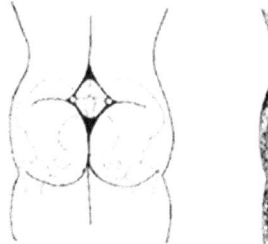

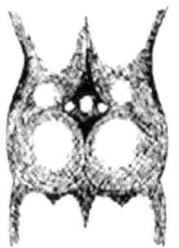

Images Sourced from Let Birth be Born Again by kind permission of Jean Sutton

THE SECOND OR ACTIVE STAGE OF BIRTHING

This stage is marked by full dilatation of the cervix leading to a change in the nature of the contractions: they become expulsive and the mother cannot prevent herself from squeezing the baby into the birth canal with each contraction.

There is usually a latent phase between the first and second stage, called 'transition', which can last from five minutes to two hours while the baby's head descends onto the pelvic floor, stimulating the reflex to bear down. Sometimes the mother can have a sleep during this period.

The mother may feel the need to have her bowels opened and that is normal. Some professionals may tell her to bear down into her bottom as if she were having a bowel movement, but the baby is going to be born through her vagina (birth canal) not her anus. The mother needs to listen to her body.

This stage culminates in the birth of the baby. The baby will still be attached to the placenta by the long umbilical cord, and the placenta will still be in the womb at this stage. The cutting of the cord will depend on the parent's wishes and prior needs.

This stage is the time portrayed on television and cinema as the 'pushing' time, but in reality, if all is going well, the woman's body doesn't need to be told how to give birth, and the midwife needs to know her wishes about this. This will be on the birth plan, but the midwife may need a reminder.

NON-DIRECTED PUSHING IN THE SECOND STAGE OF LABOUR

It has become accepted practice in the world of midwifery and obstetrics, to encourage mothers-to-be to actively push the baby out with each expulsive contraction during the second stage of labour.

The picture portrayed, in every film or documentary, and at practically every birth in every hospital in the western world, is of panic and noise, with everyone shouting the obligatory 'push, push, push'. The common belief amongst laypeople is that the mother has to be told, shouted at and cajoled in every way possible for the birth to take place. No one seems to know when this practice began, but probably busy doctors and midwives, in homes and hospitals, tired and with other pressures on their time, with one eye on the clock, mistakenly believing that everyone wants to see this baby because they have waited long enough, it has become ingrained in practice and everyone has followed - like sheep.

The pressure to 'push, push, push' is written in hospital protocols, with various time limits applied from the moment it is established the cervix is fully dilated. This is called the latent stage and is just when the mother needs a rest, to build up her strength for the work ahead. Some establishments and practitioners encourage the mother to start pushing immediately the cervix is deemed to be dilated, and expect the baby to be born within an hour or two, or sometimes more, depending on the protocols that apply in that particular establishment.

In addition, the mother is usually flat on her back, which is the worst possible position for giving birth (please see the chapter on Optimal Foetal Positioning).

In the worst-case scenario, the mother is made to feel guilty if she doesn't deliver within the prescribed time. Tiredness, exhaustion, and her birth attendants telling her the baby is getting tired wear down her resistance and patience, and if forceps are suggested or, even in extreme circumstances, a caesarean section is considered, she is likely to agree to anything.

Sadly, her feelings afterwards may be of guilt because she has been made to feel she did not try hard enough. That's not fair! She deserves a medal for all her efforts. Actually, during the expulsive stage of labour, the mother couldn't stop pushing if she tried, which says everything.

Knowledge and common sense are finally beginning to grow in the field of aiming for a natural birth, and some research has taken place, with papers published on the negative effects of directed pushing on mother and baby, and even the dangers of this method. Not allowing all the structures in the birth canal to slowly stretch to allow the baby to pass gently into the world can have harmful effects on the pelvic floor.

There is evidence of other harmful effects of this type of management of the second stage of labour, but it is not the purpose of this book to frighten expectant parents but to point the reader in the direction of having the best possible chance of a natural and pleasant experience when it comes to the birth of their baby.

If we observe animals, they go to a quiet, dark, and safe place, away from danger and do not need directions of any kind to give birth, especially being directed to push. Of course, we are human, and for wild animals, there is no one there to intervene when the occasional need arises.

We must not get carried away and presume that intervention is never necessary. When there are genuine signs of problems, of course, with adequate explanation, all available medical help must be accepted.

However, non-directed pushing, when the mother is relaxed and allowing her body to work as it is intended, allowing the expulsive contractions to take place in their own time may take longer, but it is a much safer and happier birth for all concerned.

RESOURCES:

MIDWIFE-LED CONTINUITY MODELS OF CARE COMPARED WITH OTHER

www.cochrane.org/CD004667/PREG_midwife-led-continuity-models-care-compared-other-models-care-women-during-pregnancy-birth-and-early

Women who had midwife-led continuity models of care were more likely to experience no intrapartum analgesia/anaesthesia…, have a longer mean length of labour … and more likely to be attended at birth by a known midwife...

RECOMMENDATIONS | INTRAPARTUM CARE FOR HEALTHY WOMEN

nice.org.uk/guidance/cg190/chapter/recommendations

Women who are receiving midwifery-led care in an obstetric unit can have their care transferred to obstetric-led care without being moved. 1.6.1 Base any decisions about transfer of care on clinical findings, and discuss the options with the woman and her birth companion(s).

SUPPORTING WOMEN'S INSTINCTIVE PUSHING BEHAVIOUR DURING BIRTH

https://midwifethinking.com/2015/09/09/supporting-womens-instinctive-pushing-behaviour-during-birth/

09/09/2015 Directed pushing was introduced in an attempt to shorten the duration of the 'second stage of labour' in the belief that this would improve outcomes for women and babies (Bosomworth and Bettany-Saltikov 2006).

WHEN AND HOW TO PUSH: PROVIDING THE MOST CURRENT INFORMATION.

https://www.ncbi.nlm.nih.gov/pmc/articles/PMC1804305/

By KR Simpson - 2006 - Cited by 14 Related articles

EFFECT OF THE TYPE OF MATERNAL PUSHING DURING THE SECOND STAGE OF...

https://bmjopen.bmj.com/content/6/12/e012290

By C Barasinski - 2016 - Cited by 3 Related articles

The objective of our study is to assess and compare the effectiveness of directed closed-glottis (Valsalva) pushing (pushing while holding one's breath) versus directed open-glottis pushing (pushing during a prolonged exhalation), during the second stage of labour.

THE THIRD STAGE OF LABOUR

The birth of the placenta (afterbirth), and the time it takes, will depend on whether the physiological (natural) third stage is planned or is managed with the aid of the drug Syntometrine, as explained in the section 'Active Management of the Third Stage of Labour' further along in this book.

THE DIFFERENCE BETWEEN A NATURAL AND MANAGED THIRD STAGE

After the birth of the baby, the mother needs to stay relaxed to allow the placenta (afterbirth) to come away. Women can choose the way the afterbirth/placenta is born whether in hospital or home. This is called the 'third stage of labour'.

There have been many studies of the best way to deal with the third stage of birth but, in the end, it is the woman's choice, and with the benefit of knowledge she can make an informed choice.

If the third stage is managed, it means an injection of Syntometrine is given in the thigh at the point of birth, although the woman may not even be aware of it unless she is told at the time it is given, or before the birth. The injection is to aid the expulsion of the placenta, and the midwife should explain its action, and the reason, it is offered well before the birth so that consent, if it is given, is understood and informed.

RESOURCES

DELIVERING THE PLACENTA IN THE THIRD STAGE OF LABOUR | COCHRANE

www.cochrane.org/CD007412/PREG_delivering-placenta-third-stage-labour

THIRD STAGE OF LABOUR: DELIVERING PLACENTA AND CORD CLAMPING

www.nct.org.uk/labour-birth/your-guide-labour/third-stage-labour-delivering-placenta-and-cord-clamping

The third stage of labour is the time between when you have your baby and when the placenta (or afterbirth) comes out. (Begley et al, 2011; NICE, 2017). Once your baby's born, the release of the hormone oxytocin will make the uterus contract and become smaller. This will then make the placenta start to separate.

THE THIRD STAGE OF LABOUR: ACTIVE OR EXPECTANT MANAGEMENT OF

www.evidentlycochrane.net/third-stage-of-labour

29/08/2019 ·Two approaches to care in the third stage.

Care during the third stage of labour (from the birth of the baby to the birth of the placenta and membranes) remains an issue for debate among women and practitioners on the optimum method of management.

PHYSIOLOGICAL THIRD STAGE

If a natural or physiological third stage is chosen, no drugs are given and it can take about thirty minutes (but *can* take one to two hours) for the placenta to separate and come away; it is not painful.

The uterus will contract with expulsive contractions, but not as strong as those felt during the birth, and skin-to-skin contact with baby and breastfeeding can help this process.

The woman will feel gentle, pushing urges, and gradually, after some contractions, the placenta slides out. This is the end of the third stage of labour (birthing) and is the end of the period when the baby is dependent on the placenta for oxygen and nutrients from the mother's blood.

In a physiological third stage, the umbilical cord is not cut until it has stopped pulsating. This is to allow the maximum amount of blood from the placenta to reach the baby. There are many benefits to this, such as a reduced risk of anaemia after birth. This is discussed later in the chapter on delayed cord clamping.

During this stage, the baby's lungs inflate and breathing commences naturally.

The umbilical cord is clamped in two places and the cord is then cut between the two clamps. Some parents may wish to see the placenta; if so, the midwife will be happy to show it to them.

There is a greater loss of blood with a natural third stage of labour, and the professionals who favour this method say that a blood loss of 500 ml or more is normal. They say that this is nature's way of dealing with the physiological needs of the mother following the birth of her baby. Therefore, when choosing between a physiological or managed third stage of labour, consideration needs to be given to the following:

- The length of time of the labour.

- How much intervention was undertaken and the reasons for this.

- And importantly, how experienced and knowledgeable about the natural third stages of birth are the professionals attending the birth.

In the unusual event of the third stage being prolonged, or if blood loss is excessive, the drug Ergometrine is used, via a vein in the back of the hand, which acts to control the bleeding by stimulating the uterus to contract and expel the placenta in seconds. Unless it is an emergency there is usually time for explanations to be given.

Historically, this has been the most dangerous phase of childbirth and, in past times, post-partum haemorrhage (excessive bleeding after the birth of a baby) was a common cause of maternal death. Countless lives have been saved by the use of drugs such as oxytocin and Ergometrine. These two drugs are combined in Syntometrine, which is commonly used in the UK, and in other countries, the same drugs will have a different name.

The uterus will continue to contract for a few days after the baby is born as it begins to return to its non-pregnant size, particularly when breastfeeding, and if this feels uncomfortable (especially after your first baby) relaxation methods will help.

ACTIVE MANAGEMENT OF THE THIRD STAGE

Active management of the third stage means the administering of a drug called Syntometrine, which causes the uterus to contract rapidly between two and a half minutes and up to six or seven minutes. It is believed that this method ensures quick 'delivery' of the placenta and reduced blood loss. When this method is offered, an explanation should be given and permission obtained.

For many years, the use of these drugs became so widespread in the developed world that health professionals were not taught how to look after women during the third stage of labour without the use of the oxytocin drugs. The case is proven that using the drugs at this time reduces the amount of blood loss, but there is insufficient evidence on the adverse effects of these drugs, e.g. nausea, vomiting, headaches, and high blood pressure.

The preference of the mother-to-be can be written on the birth plan when she has had time to consider the evidence for and against so that she is not pressurised at the point of birth. When clients are treated with respect and told what is going on, they will understand and agree when intervention is absolutely necessary, because they will trust the professionals responsible for their care.

The injection causes the uterus to contract more strongly to enable the placenta to separate more quickly. The midwife gently pulls on the cord as the uterus contracts, until the placenta and membranes come away, and pushing is not required. This called Controlled Cord Traction.

DELAYED CORD CLAMPING (DCC)

It is common practice, in birthing establishments everywhere, to cut the umbilical cord, which connects the placenta to the baby, immediately after birth, especially when an injection of Syntometrine (this is explained in 'Active Management of the Third Stage') has been given, thus cutting off the baby's supply of blood and oxygen, which has been sustaining it for the duration of the pregnancy.

The effect of this is that the baby is deprived of thirty per cent of the blood volume he would have received if the birth attendants had waited until the cord had stopped pulsating. Evidence shows that immediate cord clamping can deprive the foetus of up to 214 g of cord blood, equating to approximately thirty per cent of their intended blood volume (Farrer 2010). As soon as the cord is cut the baby is forced to breathe, as his oxygen supply has been cut off (also explained in the chapter 'Physiological Third Stage of Labour').

Requesting delayed cord clamping on your birth plan is very important if that is per your wishes. Bear in mind that there are circumstances during the birth when it might be necessary for reasons not to wait, which your birth attendants should have a good explanation for. We must always be sensible and accept when intervention is essential for the well-being of mother and baby.

Ola Anderson, 2011, carried out an RCT (random controlled trial) which showed that babies who had immediate cord clamping (ICC) had higher incidences of iron deficiency anaemia at four months of age.

Judith Mercer, a Professor of Midwifery in the USA, has done extensive research showing that premature babies benefit more from DCC and have less incidence of intraventricular haemorrhage and necrotising enterocolitis. Judith Mercer recommends that all babies have cord clamping delayed for at least five minutes.

Resources:

Quality Statement 6: Delayed Cord Clamping | Intrapartum Care

www.nice.org.uk/guidance/qs105/chapter/quality-statement-6-delayed-cord-clamping

10/12/2015 ·Women do not have the cord clamped earlier than 1 minute after the birth unless there is concern about cord integrity or the baby's heartbeat. Rationale The Benefits of delayed cord clamping

includes higher haemoglobin concentrations, a decreased risk of iron deficiency and greater vascular stability in babies.

Latest recommendations on timing of clamping the umbilical cord

www.researchgate.net/publication/281459462_Latest_recommendations_on_timing_of_clamping_the_umbilical_cord

Latest recommendations on the timing of clamping the umbilical cord The RCM are very engaged with members who are currently moving forward with their own Better Births initiatives at a local level.

Delaying the clampers | AIMS

www.aims.org.uk/journal/item/delaying-the-clampers

Amanda Burleigh explains the call to change NICE guidance on cord clamping. Approximately 50 years ago oxytocic drugs were introduced to labouring women to shorten the third stage of labour, preventing postpartum haemorrhage and improving the mortality rate. The function of the umbilical cord was not even considered, never mind researched, and immediate clamping and cutting became standard practice, often occurring before the baby had taken its first breath.

THE PLACENTA (AFTERBIRTH)

The baby was dependent on the placenta for oxygen and nutrients from the mother's blood.

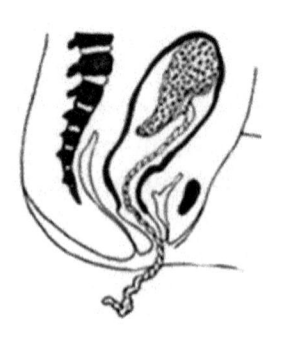

The placenta after the birth of the baby when the umbilical cord has been cut.

The placenta is an amazing organ that sustains the foetus during the pregnancy; it is attached to the wall of the womb and it provides the baby with blood from your blood supply (although the two blood supplies are separate). The placenta provides your unborn baby with all the nutrients and oxygen they need, protects against infection, produces hormones to support the pregnancy, and removes waste products from the baby's blood. The umbilical cord arises from the placenta and is the link between mother and baby.

It is well-known that most animals eat the placenta, and it has become popular for some mothers to believe that eating the placenta, or part of it, would be beneficial - to help them recover from the birth, by providing iron and essential hormones, to encourage breastmilk production, prevent infection, and possibly prevent postnatal depression. Some women have been known to eat parts of the placenta raw, or cooked and eaten with vegetables, such is the belief in its benefits.

Animals may eat the placenta to avoid attracting predators during the vulnerable time during and after birth. Some primitive and other cultures are also known to favour eating the placenta, and this could be for the same reason - in our genes from way back in our history.

PLACENTAL ENCAPSULATION

It is believed that the nutrients and hormones that have sustained the foetus may be beneficial for the mother to ingest, as most other mammals do, and which it is claimed will, amongst other attributes, relieve pain, and help with bonding and breastfeeding. To make ingestion of the placenta easier, a method of drying it and putting it into capsules has been devised as a more palatable way of receiving the benefits it is believed to offer.

Placental encapsulation has become so popular now that training is provided for those going into the placental encapsulation business. Information packs are provided antenatally, and a collection and delivery service provided.

There is no evidence to support the eating of the placenta or the consumption of the capsules; however, there is anecdotal evidence that the capsules could be a source of infection, and could harm the mother and, through the breast milk, the baby.

Whatever your beliefs, it is wise to research this practice as much as possible to protect you and your baby.

Resources:

The Evidence on Placenta Encapsulation

https://evidencebasedbirth.com/evidence-on-placenta-encapsulation/

22/02/2017 · Human placenta processed for encapsulation contains modest concentrations of 14 trace minerals and elements. Nutrition Research 36(8): 872-8. Young, S. M., Gryder, L. K., Zava, D., et al. (2016). Presence and concentration of 17 hormones in the human placenta processed for encapsulation and consumption. Placenta 43: 86-9.

What are the benefits and risks of eating placenta?

https://www.medicalnewstoday.com/articles/319806

19/10/2017 · The practice of eating placenta, or "placentophagy," is common in the animal kingdom. It is believed that most non-human mammals with a placenta consume their "afterbirth" – as the placenta is...

Eating the Placenta: A Good Idea? - Mayo Clinic

www.mayoclinic.org/healthy-lifestyle/labor-and-delivery/expert-answers/eating-the-placenta/faq-20380880

16/08/2019 · The most common placenta preparation – creating a capsule – is made by steaming and dehydrating the placenta or processing the raw placenta. People have also been known to eat the placenta raw, cooked, or in smoothies or liquid extracts.

THE BABY

APGAR SCORE

The Apgar score was invented by anaesthetist Virginia Apgar in 1952 and is the respected current routine practice, still used worldwide, to evaluate the newborn at the moment of birth. It is a very painless, simple and effective check made on the baby by midwives and doctors to assess the baby's health and is a guide to refer to later.

      One minute after birth and again five minutes later, the midwife and doctor will assess the baby's condition and the resulting score will be used to decide whether the baby needs any immediate treatment. The score is from 0 to 10, is non-invasive and causes no disturbance to mother or baby.

ACRONYM	SCORE OF 0	SCORE OF 1	SCORE OF 2
SKIN COLOUR	BLUE ALL OVER	WHITE AT EXTREMITIES BODY PINK	PINK ALL OVER
HEART RATE	ABSENT	SLOW	FAST
REFLEX RESPONSE	NO RESPONSE TO STIMULATION	GRIMACING WHEN STIMULATED	CRYING AND COUGHING
MUSCLE TONE	LIMP	SOME BENDING OR STRETCHING OF LIMBS	ACTIVE MOVEMENT
BREATHING	ABSENT	WEAK OR IRREGULAR	GOOD AND YOUR BABY IS CRYING

Most newborns have a score between 7 and 10, and if your baby has a low score the check will be made over and over until it has settled to a higher score.

RESOURCES:

APGAR SCORE - BABYCENTRE UK

www.babycentre.co.uk/a3074/apgar-score

Apgar Score: Chart, Definition, Normal, Baby, and More
www.healthline.com/health/apgar-score

The Apgar score is a scoring system doctors and nurses use to assess newborns one minute and five minutes after they're born. Dr. Virginia Apgar created the system in 1952 and used her name as a mnemonic... Author: Rachel Nall, MSN, CRNA

VERNIX CASEOSA

This is a white, creamy substance covering the baby during the last trimester of pregnancy. It provides a waterproof covering for the skin as the baby is immersed in the fluid and protects it from infection whilst in the womb. The amount reduces closer to the due date, so early babies have quite a thick covering but by term, it is almost all absorbed.

As well as protection whilst in the womb, the vernix acts as a lubricant in its journey through the birth canal, and after the birth, the beneficial properties continue. It contains antimicrobial and anti-inflammatory properties giving protection from infection, moisturises the skin, contains antioxidants and is believed to help regulate the baby's temperature. It is well to consider leaving the vernix on and delaying bathing the baby until it has been absorbed, so your baby can benefit from all that it provides and has that lovely soft skin after birth.

RESOURCES:

VERNIX CASEOSA: BENEFITS FOR BABY - HEALTHLINE

www.healthline.com/health/pregnancy/vernix-caseosa

16/06/2016 The vernix caseosa is a protective layer on your baby's skin. It appears as a white, cheese-like substance. This coating develops on the baby's skin while in the womb. Traces of the substance may appear on the skin after birth. Author: Valencia Higuera

VITAMIN K

Vitamin K is a component that helps with the clotting of blood. There is a rare condition affecting newborn babies called Haemorrhagic Disease of the Newborn, caused by insufficient vitamin K. This affects a very small number, about 1 in 10,000 of babies who don't have enough vitamin K to help their blood clot, which can result in spontaneous bruising or a bleed. It can happen within twelve weeks after birth.

In the UK, parents are routinely asked if they wish their babies to have vitamin K by mouth or intramuscular injection. It is a generally accepted policy, in the care of the newborn, to administer vitamin K to all babies soon after birth as a precautionary measure. The best method of vitamin administration is by intramuscular injection into the baby's thigh (it takes a second and usually the baby hardly notices). It can be given orally, but it is less effective and may need to be given again in a few weeks.

Resources:

Vitamin K - BabyCentre UK

www.babycentre.co.uk/a551938/vitamin-k

Vitamin K (Konakion MM) For Babies - Information For Parents - NHS

www.hey.nhs.uk/patient-leaflet/vitamin-k-konakion-mm-babies-information-parents/

This is recommended by The Department of Health in the UK

Vitamin K: Injection or Oral Dose for Newborns | NCT

https://www.nct.org.uk/parenting/vitamin-k

Injections after birth - what did YOU do? | Mumsnet

Vitamin K? | Netmums

www.netmums.com/coffeehouse/becoming-mum-pregnancy-996/netmums-52/699736-vitamin-k.html

In my hospital notes on my labour and birth plan page, it asks: Would I like my baby to have Vitamin K?

EXAMINATION OF THE NEWBORN

As soon as reasonably possible after birth, your new baby will be weighed, and you will be anxious to know the weight. It is also an important part of the first health assessment of your baby. Measurements of the circumference of the head and sometimes the length are also taken. The midwife or paediatrician will also do a thorough head-to-toe examination, the details of which are beyond the scope of this book but include examining the skull, eyes, ears, mouth, heart, hips, and in boys, the testes.

The examination should be carried out in the presence of the parents and a full explanation given for each part of the examination. All the findings are documented and repeated on discharge from the hospital, and by the GP at the 6-week postnatal check. Any relevant findings are discussed with the parents.

RESOURCES:

NEWBORN PHYSICAL EXAMINATION - **NHS**

WWW.NHS.UK/CONDITIONS/PREGNANCY-AND-BABY/NEWBORN-PHYSICAL-EXAM/

During the examination, the health professional will also: look into your baby's eyes with a special torch to check how their eyes look and move, listen to your baby's heart to check their heart sounds, examine their hips to check the joints, and examine baby boys to see if their testicles have descended.

EXAMINATION OF THE NEWBORN: THE FIRST 72 HOURS OF LIFE

www.ausmed.com/cpd/articles/examination-of-the-newborn/

The Newborn Examination: Observe the baby's general condition, including colour, breathing, behaviour, activity, posture and cry. Head and skull. Note facial symmetry, the size of the fontanelles and the presence of any remaining caput, cephalhematoma or trauma. Note the position and placement of the ears.

NEWBORN COMMUNICATION

THE FIRST HOUR

After birth, the mother or parents of the baby may spend a long time gazing at each other, beginning the process of getting to know each other. The baby will recognise the mother's smell and the sound of her voice, as well as the father's if he has been communicating with the 'bump' before the birth.

The baby will communicate its need for food by the 'rooting reflex', turning its head towards the mother's breast, making mouthing movements and putting its tongue out.

In these first minutes after birth, the infant is in the 'quiet alert' state, and this ability to communicate with the mother at this time may be nature's way of preparing them for their future attachment to the mother.

The baby's irresistible, wide-eyed, appealing face will touch hearts, and the parents and baby will fall in love with each other.

Slowly the parents will learn all the signs that their baby is communicating with them and they will understand its needs.

Of course, crying is the baby's most powerful form of communication. But the special quiet times when the baby is feeding or just being held, with the parents enjoying the pleasure of its presence, the baby's love will be communicated by facial expressions. They may even copy facial movements, demonstrating that this tiny bundle is acutely aware of everything that is going on.

When the mother or father instinctively look into their baby's eyes and talk 'baby talk', telling them stories and telling them how much they love them, the baby is listening to every word, fascinated by their faces and the sounds of their voices which are so familiar.

Talk to the baby all the time, play soft music and sing to them. Toys are not necessary for the first few weeks; the baby only needs its mother or father. Even if they are just sitting quietly gazing at their baby, s/he will feel the security of their love.

At around the age of six weeks or so something magical will happen and the baby will smile. At first, it will be fleeting, but they will have been practising beforehand, and when it happens, there is no mistaking that the smile is especially for the person it is looking at, as the whole face and eyes will smile straight back.

These smiles will become longer and more frequent until they become gurgles and later hearty laughs.

When the baby is tired they will turn away. It is its way of saying the conversation is over for now because a baby's attention span is short in the early weeks. The baby can 'switch off' when tired or overstimulated.

This is the wonderful newborn that loves and needs you, and all this love and communication began in the months before he was born.

THE NEWBORN BABY

Babies are born with a very strong instinct to survive. Two very powerful examples are the sucking reflex and crying.

Following an uncomplicated birth, the newborn baby, if given the opportunity, and if placed prone on the mother's abdomen, will find the breast and the nipple and commence to suckle without assistance, thus obtaining the very important colostrum and stimulating the mother's breasts to continue the process of lactation, providing the perfect food at each feed and each stage in the baby's growth.

Growth during the first three months of the baby's life is faster than at any other time in their life and is comparable with the growth pattern of puberty. It is a critical stage for the development of the digestive system and the brain.

The first cry of a newborn baby occurs after birth when the umbilical cord is cut making it necessary for the baby to breathe to obtain oxygen, previously obtained via the placenta. The change in temperature from the warmth of the womb into the outside air (even when warmed) will stimulate the baby to cry.

When the birth and third stage (the birth of

the placenta) is natural and unaided by synthetic hormones, and the umbilical cord is not cut until it has finished pulsating, the changeover from oxygen from the placenta to oxygen from the air is gradual, allowing the lungs to inflate slowly instead of suddenly as when the cord is cut whilst still pulsating and receiving blood and oxygen from the placenta.

From this time the baby's cries are an alarm signal to the mother if he/she feels insecure, such as feeling alone and vulnerable, hungry, uncomfortable, or in pain or discomfort for any reason.

Crying is the baby's communication system for survival. He/she has no concept of time, their need is immediate and, until the cries are answered, feels abandoned and exposed to danger, which is a primitive response.

Prolonged crying produces the stress hormone cortisol, which is known in excess, to cause emotional harm to the brain. Parents who believe they are training their newborn by leaving them to cry and wait for attention or feeding, are unaware that the reason the baby eventually stops crying is that it learns that no one is going to come, and the baby goes into a deep traumatised sleep, thus reinforcing the parent's belief that the baby has been trained to settle.

In these first few months of life, the baby needs the closeness, warmth and security of a human body and to hear the reassuring voices that have been heard whilst in the womb. Gradually, during these early weeks and months, the baby can be put down in a pram or cot and learn to lie happily awake or to settle to sleep when tired, provided all nutritional needs have been met and there are no other discomforts.

This baby will be secure and emotionally balanced, and by approximately three months or so will happily go down in his/her cot in the evening, after a bath or feed, and self-settle for twelve hours' sleep.

Bedtime should be a calm time without too much stimulation or excitement, leading to a happy bedtime, with a story later as they grow into a child.

STEM CELLS

Stem cells are in our bodies all of our lives. They are primal cells, and allow our body to heal and repair damaged tissue such as muscle and broken bones; they are continually working to replace worn-out and damaged specialised parts of our bodies. Research is ongoing to understand how stem cells can be used to find and develop new treatments for many different diseases.

At present (2020) only bone marrow transplants are medically approved for the use of stem cells in the United Kingdom, for treating immune system and blood disorders.

Although not for general use, other stem cell treatments are being researched in clinical trials in the UK, e.g. for skin grafts, the cornea of the eye damage, and others, some showing promise and hope for the future.

STEM CELLS FROM UMBILICAL CORD BLOOD

Blood taken from the umbilical cord soon after birth is a rich source of stem cells, the ultimate repair kit.

In recent years, expectant parents have considered obtaining their baby's cord blood in the hope that, in the future, should the child develop an illness for which the stem cell treatment is appropriate, the stored cord blood could be used. Several private companies are being contracted to do this, and these companies have to be accredited by the Human Tissue

Authority (HTA) and the Medical and Healthcare Products Regulatory Agency (MHRA).

The companies offering this service provide a collection kit and an assigned health professional trained to carry out the procedure. The blood is then transferred to the specialised blood bank by courier. The procedure takes about ten minutes, is painless for you and your baby, and is non-invasive to you both.

If your birth is in hospital, permission is necessary from the hospital authorities, and it is also important to inform all your professional carers to ensure it is on your birth plan and your antenatal notes.

RESOURCES:

CORD BLOOD BANKING: A GUIDE FOR PARENTS | HUMAN TISSUE AUTHORITY

https://www.hta.gov.uk/guidance-public/cord-blood-banking-guide-parents

You need to know your rights and options regarding the facts on umbilical cord blood banking when dealing with the HTA.

EUROSTEMCELL | MEDIA AND RESOURCE LIBRARY

www.eurostemcell.org

Unapproved stem cell treatments are sometimes offered by unregulated companies and clinics.

Unapproved procedures often lack scientific evidence showing they work and may even be dangerous. Patients must discuss medical decisions with their GP before seeking out medical treatments.

Umbilical Cord Blood: Current Status and Future Directions - McKenna

https://onlinelibrary.wiley.com/doi/abs/10.1111/j.1423-0410.2010.01409.x

By DH McKenna - 2011 - Cited by 35 - Related articles 22 Dec 2010 - Once considered biological waste, umbilical cord blood (UCB) has become an accepted source of haematopoietic stem cells (HSCs).

Future Health Biobank: Private Stem Cell Banking and Genetic Screening

https://futurehealthbiobank.com/

Future Health Biobank. The UK's stem cell bank. Offering umbilical cord blood & tissue stem cell banking.

AFTER THE BIRTH

THE FIRST HOUR

Michel Odent, who is the founder of the Centre for Primal Research in London, advocates natural childbirth with minimum intervention and the critical importance of the first hour after birth, for the benefit of mother and baby.

It is common practice in hospitals, to take the baby to a special trolley, which is kept in the birthing room, in the belief that it may need help warming up after birth. This trolley has an overhead heater and other equipment to give any care the baby may need, with the baby being returned as soon as possible.

In reality, the best place to warm the newborn is skin-to-skin on the mother's body; in fact, there are several reasons why? Ideally, the only person who should hold the baby is the mother. The baby's skin is sterile, but within the first hour it is colonised by millions of bacteria (as we all are), and as mother and baby share the same antibodies, the mother's skin is the best environment for the baby. Breathing becomes established as the baby's lungs adjust to receiving oxygen from the air instead of the placenta. This is also the special bonding time when the mother's hormone, oxytocin, will be at its highest, helping the birth of the placenta, and the initiation of breastfeeding. The mother must not be distracted during this special, quiet, peaceful time.

Soon the baby will start 'rooting' for the breast, and feeding will help to assist the birth of the placenta if it has not already happened. The first breastfeed is most important and an alert baby (one who has not been affected by medication given to the mother during the labour) will find the breast and latch on to the nipple unaided, thus receiving the vitally important first feed of colostrum, and gaining the best possible protection with the natural gut flora and antibodies. The colostrum also supplies the essential glucose, which will be low at this point since the baby's supply of glucose from the placenta has stopped. The new mother and her partner will also appreciate some time together on their own.

In unavoidable circumstances, it may be necessary to disturb this process, always bearing in mind that the best interests of mother and baby must be paramount, for the baby to be taken to the trolley for treatment. The parents will want to welcome their baby into the world in their way, but in this case, the parents need to trust professional people to take care of the baby. Usually, the midwife will give them both refreshments of their choice.

Eventually, depending on hospital protocols, the baby will be weighed, and a routine examination carried out. If all is well, and it is the parent's choice, they may be discharged from the hospital within a few hours of the birth.

When they arrive home they should try to maintain a calm atmosphere. Delay the rush of visitors for a while. The parents will be feeling tired and so will their baby. They all need bonding and resting time.

Resources:

Michel Odent and the First Hour of Life – Mary-Rose MacColl

www.mary-rosemaccoll.com/blog/2013/1/14/michel-odent-and-the-first-hour-of-life

14 Jan 2013 - French obstetrician Michel Odent has spent the last several decades trying to make the world think about the importance of birth.

The First Hour Following Birth: Don't Wake the Mother! By Michel Odent | Midwifery Today

https://midwiferytoday.com/mt-articles/first-hour/

1 Mar 2002 - It is well understood that during the first hour following birth the baby must suddenly use its lungs.

Fathers: Those Engrossing First Minutes | Midwifery Today

https://midwiferytoday.com/mt-articles/fathers-engrossing-first-minutes

Later, long hours together spent cuddling and playing will help mould a permanent tie that they will depend on throughout life.

WHEN COMPLICATIONS HAPPEN

PRETERM BIRTH

A spontaneous or elective birth between twenty-four and thirty-seven weeks of gestation is considered preterm. At twenty-four weeks gestation, the foetus is considered 'viable', which is capable of surviving outside the womb. Of course, the closer to twenty-four weeks the more vulnerable the baby will be, and the more medical care and support will be required.

The closer to thirty-seven weeks, as more development and growth has taken place, the less specialised care will be needed, and very often baby can be discharged home, requiring careful observation and frequent feeds until the baby has reached a stable weight gain.

Very early babies require care in a specialised neonatal unit, possibly ventilated in an incubator to help with breathing as the lungs will be immature. Other support will be given, such as nutrition via a nasal tube or intravenously, temperature control and all the baby's vital signs will be constantly monitored by specially trained nursing staff. The parents will be encouraged to see their baby as soon as possible and will be helped to touch and hold their baby, even help with feeding, whenever this is safe and medically possible.

It is a very anxious and worrying time for new parents, especially when it has happened unexpectedly, with no preparation possible beforehand and maybe no time for antenatal classes. So parents will be very shocked and needing all the kindness and understanding from the hospital professionals, who are usually only too pleased to explain and answer questions about the baby's progress and developments as they occur.

Bliss is an organisation that gives free support and information to parents of preterm babies, with information leaflets and other methods of help. The staff caring for your baby will put you in touch with this organisation.

Babies born between twenty-two and twenty-six weeks gestation can still survive, but will be classed as 'extremely preterm' babies, and will need extra special care as there could be other complications.

RESOURCES:

BLISS: FOR BABIES BORN PREMATURE OR SICK

www.bliss.org.uk/

Our vision is that every baby born premature or sick in the UK has the best chance of survival and quality of life.

VIABILITY OF EXTREMELY PREMATURE BABIES | BRIEFINGS | ADVOCACY | BPAS

www.bpas.org/get-involved/advocacy/briefings/premature-babies/

SMALL-FOR-DATES BABY

Sometimes although not born before their due day, babies can have some problems affecting growth in the womb and be born smaller than expected for the EDD. They may need similar help as the preterm babies in the neonatal unit.

It may be necessary to induce labour early if the baby is perceived to be at risk or the mother's health is causing concern.

POST-TERM

Pregnancy is meant to last forty weeks, and post-term pregnancy is usually defined as ten days after the estimated date of delivery. However, this can be a controversial topic amongst obstetricians, midwives and others, as it is only an estimated date, and some practitioners consider that as long as both the mother and the baby are well, induction should be avoided if at all possible.

There has been little research on this subject and parents now have to take advice from their caregiver to decide on the management of the pregnancy when it has gone overdue according to the guidelines.

RESOURCES:

Women's Experiences and Attitudes Towards Expectant Management and Induction of Labour in Post-term Pregnancy

https://doi.org/10.1080/00016340701416929

Runa Heimstad, Pål R Romundstad, Jon Hyett, Lars-Åke Mattson, Kjell Å Salvesen
An interesting study of 508 women. At 41 weeks 74% of women preferred induction of labour. There are differing opinions between obstetric practitioners.

Watchful Waiting or Induction of Labour – A Matter of Informed Choice: Identification, Analysis and Critical Appraisal of Decision Aids and Patient Information Regarding Care Options for Women with Uncomplicated Singleton Late and Post-term Pregnancies: A Review.

https://pubmed.ncbi.nlm.nih.gov/25947100/
Source: PubMed – 07 May 2015 – Publisher: Bmc Complementary and Alternative Medicine

MALPRESENTATIONS (BREECH POSITION ETC.)

When the foetus is not in the normal head-down (cephalic presentation) it is a malpresentation. Very often a malpresentation can move before labour begins and the mother can go on to have a normal birth. Other malpresentations' can be persistent and need intervention to manage and ensure a safe birth for mother and baby.

Probably the most recognisable malpresentation is breech presentation, meaning the baby is presenting bottom, feet or foot down, instead of head first.

In the past, breech births were managed by doctors or midwives, but in the present day, it is more usual for babies in this position to be born in a hospital, most likely by caesarean section. The baby may have a slightly sore bottom or maybe perfectly alright but might keep his hips flexed and be in the 'frog' position after birth. This quickly becomes more normal as the baby's kicking movements exercise the legs to straighten them out.

Other malpresentations include the occiput posterior position, meaning the baby's back is on the mother's back. This can result in a long and sometimes painful labour. Frequently, the baby changes position before or during labour.

Rare malposition's are best excluded from this book as it would only give cause for unnecessary anxiety in the reader, although a caesarean section would be necessary. Medical books and books on obstetrics are many and voluminous, and one cannot portray every possibility. Luckily, they are rare occurrences and an explanation from your professional carer will reassure you in the unlikely event that it should be necessary.

MEDICAL ASSISTANCE

MULTIPLE BIRTHS

When it is discovered that there is more than one baby it can come as a shock, which soon becomes a joy, but, depending on how many babies, it will be obvious that some extra antenatal care will be necessary.

The expectant mother of twins or more will be under the care of the consultant obstetrician, and will probably have more appointments than with a singleton pregnancy, to ensure that mother and babies have all appropriate care.

At one time, twins or even triplets were delivered at home or hospital, sometimes by the GP or midwife, naturally and without intervention. These days it is more usual for the births to take place in the hospital, and frequently by caesarean section. The mother may stay a little longer in hospital, depending on the babies' weights and to help with breastfeeding.

Multiple births are often early, which will mean more care will be needed with the babies needing to be cared for in a special neonatal unit.

RESOURCES:

TAMBA HEALTH PROFESSIONALS - NHS ENGLAND

www.england.nhs.uk/signuptosafety/wp-content/uploads/sites/16/2015/11/tamba-health-professionals-cpd.pdf

To access any of the above services please email support-team@tamba.org.uk

Your guide to Tamba – the Twins and Multiple Births

www.madeformums.com/pregnancy/your-guide-to-tamba-the-twins-and-multiple-births-association/

How Tamba was set up "It was set up by and for parents of twins, triplets and more, over 30 years ago," explains Keith Reed. "Leaders of local twins clubs decided that they needed a national organising body to help them co-ordinate their efforts and give them a much louder voice."

Twins Trust – We support twins, triplets and more

https://twinstrust.org/

Contact Twins Trust. We love hearing from you. Get in touch with Twins Trust today. Call us on 01252 332344 or contact us online.

The Multiple Births Foundation – A vital resource

www.multiplebirths.org.uk/

The Multiple Births Foundation was founded in 1988 and has become a national and international authority on multiple births.

We are the only charity internationally which employs healthcare professionals dedicated to supporting multiple birth families and educating and advising professionals about their special needs.

JANE DENTON - SCHOOL OF HEALTH SCIENCES | BIRMINGHAM CITY

www.bcu.ac.uk/health-sciences/business-and-innovation/partnership-opportunities/ebmbc/centre-staff/jane-denton

Jane Denton is Director of the Multiple Births Foundation (MBF), a charity which was founded by Dr Elizabeth Bryan, a former President of ISTS. The MBF works with professionals to raise awareness and improve services to meet the specific and special needs of multiple birth families. Jane Denton's professional background is nursing and midwifery with a specialist interest in infertility.

FORCEPS

Forceps are instruments specially designed to be used by a highly trained obstetrician, to assist the birth of the baby should there be a problem when either the position of the baby's head is delaying the process, or the baby or mother is becoming very tired, compromising the health of either or both.

The forceps are in two separate pieces, called blades, enabling the practitioner to gently apply them to either side of the baby's head, to reposition the baby's head or support the head to help lift it out of the pelvis during the mother's contractions, to birth the baby. Sometimes there may be marks on the baby's face or head due to the slight pressure from the forceps, but the marks disappear in a few days.

Should it be necessary for you to have your baby's birth assisted by forceps the professionals attending you will be able to explain in more detail with their knowledge of your particular circumstances? A local anaesthetic is given to numb the vagina before the forceps are inserted.

EPISIOTOMY

The perineum is the area of skin between the anus and the vagina, which, helped by the hormone relaxin, stretches during birth to allow the head and body of the baby to emerge. If the area is tight and delaying the birthing progress, a surgical cut is made in this area, just enough to increase the space to give the baby's head more room.

In the past, an episiotomy was performed routinely, but due to research by the late Sheila Kitzinger, anthropologist and author of *The Unkindest Cut*, it is now recommended that episiotomy is a procedure used only when necessary and at the discretion of the birth attendant.

The cut will be repaired with stitches made of an absorbable material that will not need to be removed. The procedure is performed at the height of a contraction when the pressure of the baby's head on the perineum numbs the area and pain is prevented. Alternatively, infiltration of a local anaesthetic numbs the area. An episiotomy will be performed for a forceps delivery, but not necessarily for a Ventouse extraction. Most commonly a tear occurs at the crowning of the head, which the mother is unaware of due to the pressure of the baby's head on the perineum.

Healing takes place in a few days, and the postnatal midwife will observe and advise on care and hygiene in the area. A small tear may be allowed to heal itself; only a larger tear is likely to need stitches. Ideally, the perineum is allowed to stretch slowly, and the perineum remains intact.

RESOURCES:

EPISIOTOMY DURING CHILDBIRTH: NOT JUST A 'LITTLE SNIP'

https://theconversation.com/episiotomy-during-childbirth-not-just-a-little-snip-36062

14/01/2015 It was not until the 1980s that women's voices were heard in research when Sheila Kitzinger undertook a study that exposed the trauma women suffered from the procedure.
'Just a little snip' was the usual comment from the midwife or obstetrician at the point of performing an episiotomy procedure. It was certainly more than that, and Sheila Kitzinger's campaign changed the medical protocol of routine episiotomy.

EPISIOTOMY: WHEN IT'S NEEDED, WHEN IT'S NOT – MAYO CLINIC

www.mayoclinic.org/healthy-lifestyle/labor-and-delivery/in-depth/episiotomy/art-20047282

25/08/2020 An episiotomy is an incision made in the perineum – the tissue between the vaginal opening and the anus – during childbirth. Although the procedure was once a routine part of childbirth, that's no longer the case. If you're planning a vaginal delivery, here's what you need to know about episiotomy and childbirth.

VENTOUSE EXTRACTION (VACUUM)

This procedure is performed for the same reasons that forceps are used.

The baby must be over thirty-five weeks gestation as before that time the skull bones are too soft for this method. Small plastic or metal cups are placed on the baby's head, and suction is applied via a tube to a suction device. The suction is applied with each pushing contraction, and the obstetrician or midwife gently pulls to aid the birth of the baby.

A bump or 'chignon' may appear on your baby's head where the cap was positioned. This is caused by fluid or some blood collecting in the tissues and should resolve in a few days. Long term there is no significance for the baby.

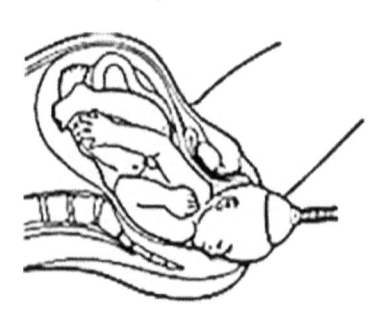

RESOURCES:

FORCEPS OR VACUUM DELIVERY - NHS

www.nhs.uk/conditions/pregnancy-and-baby/ventouse-forceps-delivery/

An assisted birth (also known as an instrumental delivery) is when forceps or a ventouse suction cup are used to help deliver the baby. Ventouse and forceps are safe and only used when necessary for you and your baby. Assisted delivery is less common in women who've had a spontaneous vaginal birth before.

FORCEPS AND VENTOUSE (ASSISTED BIRTH) - BABYCENTRE UK

www.babycentre.co.uk/a546719/forceps-and-ventouse-assisted-birth

The ventouse (vacuum extractor), has a cup attached to a suction device, and a handle to pull on. The cup fits on top and towards the back of your baby's head, and a vacuum is created within the cup. The cup is made of soft or semi-rigid plastic or metal.

OBSERVATION OF THE NEWBORN FOLLOWING VACUUM ASSISTED BIRTH [PDF]

www.slhd.nsw.gov.au/rpa/neonatal%5Ccontent/pdf/guidelines/Subgaleal.pdf

CAESAREAN SECTION

Sometimes, due to the mother's medical or obstetric history, and to ensure a healthy mother and baby, a vaginal birth will be considered undesirable, and an 'Elective Caesarean Section' will be advised. This will involve surgically removing the baby from the mother's uterus, which can be achieved under general, spinal or epidural anaesthesia.

GENERAL ANAESTHETIC

This involves being put to sleep by the anaesthetist via drugs administered through an intravenous injection and directly to the lungs via a special tube. When you wake up, your baby will be already born and presented to you as soon as possible. You will have a cannula in a vein in your hand or arm for a few hours and possibly have a urinary catheter inserted.

EPIDURAL ANALGESIA

This is a special type of pain relief which can be used in normal labour or surgery such as caesarean section. It is given by injection of a local anaesthetic in the lumbar region of the spine, in an area called the epidural space, creating numbness from the site of the injection downwards. You will be required to sit up at the side of the bed for this procedure, which can only be administered by an anaesthetist, and it usually takes a few minutes to become effective. The anaesthetist will explain in detail what is involved.

There are various levels of numbness achievable, and the appropriate level will be determined by the anaesthetist according to each situation; sometimes it is even possible to remain mobile and with an epidural catheter left in situ, so the medicine can be topped up approximately every two hours. For surgery, the numbness needs to be total, and recovery time may take a few hours after the birth. However, you will be wide awake for the birth and able to hold your baby, although it may be your partner who gets the first hold.

A screen will be set up in the operating theatre to shield the mother from seeing the operation, but she will be able to hear everything that is going on and possibly feel some pressure on the abdomen as the obstetrician and his teamwork to take the baby. The baby will be given to you as soon as possible following a quick health check. A midwife and a paediatrician will be present for each baby, especially in the case of multiple births.

An intravenous infusion will be set up to ensure that fluid levels can be monitored, and a urinary catheter is also required, as, because of the numbness, you will be unaware of the signs that the bladder is filling. Blood pressure and other vital signs will be frequently monitored.

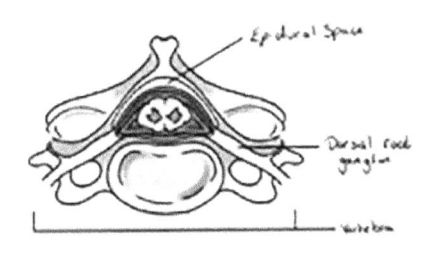

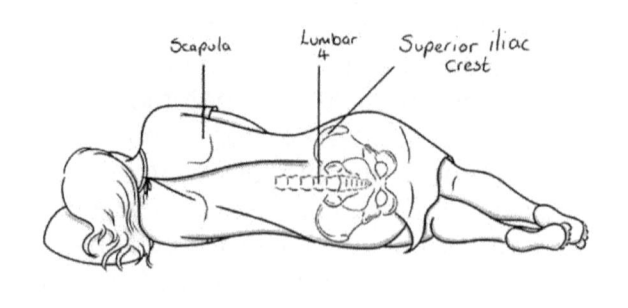

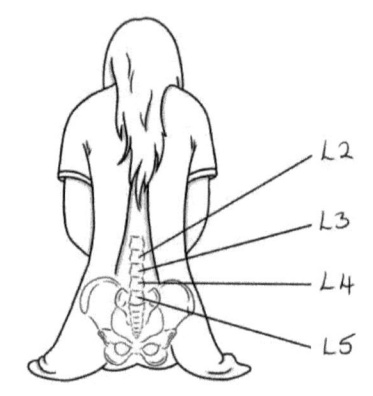

Illustrated by Laura Bagnall, Valdark Illustrations

RESOURCES:

Epidural - NHS

https://www.nhs.uk/conditions/epidural/

An epidural is an injection in the back to stop you feeling pain in part of your body.

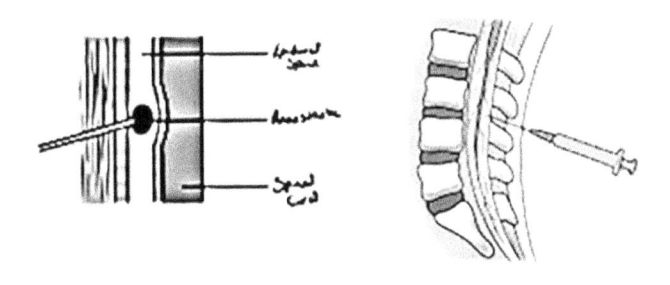

Illustrated by Laura Bagnall, Valdark Illustrations

It is easy to confuse a 'spinal block' and 'spinal epidural' because they are both injections into the spinal area. For a spinal block, narcotics or anaesthetic is injected once with a needle. For a spinal epidural or combined spinal-epidural, a catheter is placed in the epidural space to allow continuous anaesthesia.

RESOURCES:

SPINAL BLOCK - AMERICAN PREGNANCY ASSOCIATION

www.americanpregnancy.org/labor-and-birth/spinal-block

The operation will be planned in advance and the mother (and father) can be admitted to the hospital at an arranged time to prepare for the birth. It must be stated that birth by caesarean, a safe procedure these days, is a major abdominal operation and recovery time and help with breastfeeding will be necessary, as the incision area will be tender for a while.

The incision is made at the lower end of the abdomen, commonly described as the 'bikini line' and, once healed, is barely visible. This is the strongest part of the womb and is safer for future pregnancies.

The 'classical' incision is made straight down the midline of the 'bump' and is rarely used these days.

Depending on the surgeon's preference, stitches or clips will secure the incision, but both are straightforward to remove. Discharge from the hospital will depend on the condition of mother and baby but is usually in a few days.

EMERGENCY CAESAREAN SECTION

Occasionally, even when the labour appears to be progressing normally, the situation can change suddenly and, in some circumstances, an emergency caesarean will become necessary.

This can be an alarming experience. If the professional team think the health of the mother or baby might be at risk they have to act very quickly to get the baby out as soon as possible (which is their main purpose), so explanations are most important but maybe hurried and not too clear.

This is a time when you have to put your trust in the people caring for you because they are doing their best to give you the best possible chance of a happy outcome and that is what usually happens. Partners usually put on theatre dress and stay in the theatre during the operation, and will probably be the first to hold the baby. After all the anxiety, you have your baby in your arms at last.

GENTLE CAESAREAN

If you had been expecting a natural birth and, for some reason, you are advised that for medical or obstetric reasons it is best for you and your baby to have a birth by caesarean section, it is possible to request a 'gentle caesarean' which is as close as possible to vaginal delivery.

Many hospitals make this option available for mothers, but it does require forward planning and the support of the obstetric team involved. Antenatal discussions with the team are important, as this procedure takes a little more organising and time and everyone needs to be in tune with the concept and aware in advance. You may like to listen to your own music, take your own pillow or anything else familiar, to help you to be relaxed and to make this a memorable occasion.

The operating theatre is set up so that any care equipment that the baby may need after the birth is close by you, so you can see the baby at all times. Of course, hopefully, it is not needed, and your baby will be placed on your chest as the obstetric surgeon gently guides them out through the incision in your womb (uterus).

Normally a screen is placed between the mother and the operating site, but you can ask for the screen to be removed, immediately after the baby is born through the incision and placed on your chest, if that is your wish.

You will be aware of everything, and you and your partner will be more involved in the birth than when things have to be speedier, as can be essential when the caesarean is urgent.

With a gentle birth, the cord can be left intact (unless there is a reason for it to be cut) and allowed to stay so until it has stopped pulsating, as it would be in natural birth. The placenta will follow through the incision and, when ready, you can give your baby their first breastfeed.

It is important to put your desire to have a gentle caesarean on your birth plan. Discuss it with everyone on your team and ensure it is written in your patient notes, by your consultant obstetrician if possible.

Resources:

Gentle Cesarean: How To Have A More Natural C-Section

www.mamanatural.com/gentle-cesarean/

04/03/2020 · Gentle Cesarean: How to Have a More Natural C-Section 1. Implement your birth plan. Include your wishes for a gentle cesarean, even if you are planning a natural childbirth. 2. Find a doctor open to gentle c-sections. Find a doctor who is open to the idea and familiar with the concept of a gentle cesarean.

Jenny Smith - Midwife and Founder of Jentle Childbirth Foundation

https://uk.linkedin.com/in/jenny-smith-6b901646

Lectures in birth normality, nationally and internationally publications Your Body Your Baby Your Birth by Pan McMillan, midwifery and obstetric journals and media articles. Founder of Jentle Childbirth Foundation committee comprising of mothers, fathers and professional obstetricians and midwives.
Location: London, United Kingdom

MY VISIT WITH A BIRTH VISIONARY, JENNY SMITH, UK MIDWIFE | CAPPA

https://cappa.net/2020/05/18/my-visit-with-a-birth-visionary-jenny-smith-uk-midwife/

18/05/2020 · During the early 2000's, there was a growing interest in natural birth and Jenny surmised that women undergoing caesarean sections were entitled to a birth experience that could reflect some of the elements of a participatory vaginal birth. Jenny Smith assured me that this progress did not happen overnight.

JENTLE CHILDBIRTH - HOME | FACEBOOK

www.facebook.com/jentlechildbirth

Jentle Childbirth. 616 likes. The Jentle Childbirth Foundation (JCF) believes that pregnancy and childbirth should be a positive and personal experience for all women and we nurture this through. Education, training and research.
There are only two ways a baby is coming out, and it is better to plan for both options in advance.

Jentle Childbirth Foundation – Flutterby Films

https://www.flutterbyfilms.co.uk/jentle-childbirth-trust
Lovely films about all aspects of pregnancy and birth, narrated by Jenny Smith

VBAC (Vaginal Birth After Caesarean)

Sometimes, women who have had a C-section previously would like to experience a vaginal birth. In the past, women were told it was not safe to have a vaginal delivery after a caesarean section. This view applied to the classical incision, with a scar down the centre of the abdomen, (rarely, if ever, used nowadays), because there was a danger of the womb rupturing.

These days, the incision is made in the lower segment of the womb, as this is the strongest part of the womb, and it's safer to have a vaginal birth after a caesarean. The mother will be carefully monitored during the labour, with an awareness of the history and close observation of the previous scar. Records of the previous birth should be studied carefully because it has been known for an external, classical scar to be present on the abdomen and a lower-segment scar internally on the womb.

Resources:

New UK VBAC guidelines welcomed - Dr Sara Wickham

www.sarawickham.com/research-updates/new-uk-vbac-guidelines-welcomed/

01/04/2019 New UK VBAC guidelines welcomed April 1, 2019. The updated NICE guideline on Intrapartum care for women with existing medical conditions or

obstetric complications and their babies has been welcomed by midwives and other birth workers who quickly spotted changes made to the recommendations to the care offered to woman seeking a vaginal birth after a previous caesarean.

BIRTH OPTIONS AFTER A CAESAREAN SECTION | THE BMJ (BRITISH MEDICAL JOURNAL)

https://www.bmj.com/content/360/bmj.j5737
JE Norman - 2018

PREGNANCY LOSS

MISCARRIAGE

A miscarriage is when a pregnancy ends spontaneously at any time before the foetus is viable (unable to survive outside the womb), which, legally, is up to twenty-four weeks gestation. It usually occurs any time from conception, commonly around three months gestation or at eleven to thirteen weeks. The medical term for miscarriage is 'spontaneous or inevitable abortion. Statistically, it can happen in one in eight pregnancies. There are many causes, known and unknown; it can be due to the death of the embryo or foetus, or due to a defect not compatible with life.

The symptoms are cramping, abdominal discomfort and bleeding - not to be confused with the slight bleeding or 'spotting' that can occur every month during pregnancy and is common for some women. In the first few weeks of gestation, the foetus may be passed without being observed, and in later weeks a tiny foetus will be expelled.

You should contact your midwife or medical practitioner if this unfortunate event happens to you, even if you have not registered the pregnancy, as you must have a health check to ensure you have recovered medically. If you have had other miscarriages, there may need to be investigations into the possible cause and prevention for future pregnancies.

Psychologically, your loss will have a devastating effect, especially when a long-awaited baby has been planned, or even when it is unplanned. The acceptance, anticipation and preparations have begun; maybe even friends and family have been told. The impact of this early loss is bereavement and grief at the loss of a child, and how early in the pregnancy it has happened makes no difference to the extent of the grief. This was going to be your child and a part of your family.

People may not understand the impact of the loss of a baby at this stage and may make unkind and thoughtless remarks. They can be very hurtful, however unintentional and well-meant.

Counselling services, advice and support are available at this time from public-sector agencies and charity groups.

RESOURCES:

MISCARRIAGE - NHS

https://www.nhs.uk/conditions/miscarriage

The Miscarriage Association is a charity that offers support to people who have lost a baby. They have a helpline (01924 200 799, Monday to Friday, 9 am to 4 pm) and an email address (info@miscarriageassociation.org.uk), and can put you in touch with a support volunteer.

Cruse Bereavement Care helps people understand their grief and cope with their loss. They have a helpline (0808 808 1677, Monday to Friday, 9:30 am to 5 pm) and a network of local branches where you can find support.

ECTOPIC PREGNANCY

Ectopic pregnancy and loss happen when a fertilised ovum is implanted outside the womb, in one of the two fallopian tubes, and develops to the stage where it cannot survive outside the womb, becoming too large to be sustained in this environment.

Symptoms are low abdominal pain, maybe on one side, and vaginal bleeding which can be watery. Also, diarrhoea and vomiting, and pain in the tips of the shoulders can occur. This is a medical emergency requiring immediate intervention in the hospital.

Although there have been many advances in minimally invasive procedures such as keyhole surgery, it may be necessary to remove the foetus by open surgery. The fallopian tube could remain undamaged by the procedure, but in some cases, the tube might be too damaged to be saved. This does not necessarily prevent further pregnancies.

After recovery from this event, further checks and psychological support is available, as this is a very difficult, emotional and frightening event to experience.

SUPPORT GROUPS:

THE ECTOPIC PREGNANCY TRUST

http://www.ectopic.org.uk/

THE ECTOPIC PREGNANCY FOUNDATION

http://www.ectopicpregnancy.co.uk/

ECTOPIC PREGNANCY - NHS

www.nhs.uk/conditions/Ectopic-pregnancy/

An ectopic pregnancy is when a fertilised egg implants itself outside of the womb, usually in one of the fallopian tubes. The fallopian tubes are the tubes connecting the ovaries to the womb. If an egg gets stuck in them, it won't develop into a baby and your health may be at risk if the pregnancy continues.

THE MISCARRIAGE ASSOCIATION

http://www.miscarriageassociation.org.uk/

CRUSE BEREAVEMENT CARE

http://www.cruse.org.uk/

LATE MISCARRIAGE

This can happen as the pregnancy progresses, up to twenty-four weeks gestation or mid-2nd trimester, when the foetus is growing and developing more and more into a recognisable small baby; this comes as a huge shock.

At a time when the pregnancy has seemingly passed the risk of miscarriage, it is very distressing, physically and emotionally.

If contractions start at this stage and birth appears to be imminent, it is obvious that, if the baby is born, it is not sufficiently developed to sustain life outside the womb. Sometimes this is inevitable, but in some circumstances, it may be possible to save the pregnancy and to go on to full term.

There are instances of survival below the twenty-four-week gestation, at which point they become legally considered viable, but this is rare and requires exceptional circumstances and a very long period in the neonatal intensive care unit with expert, devoted care and attention.

Help is available should you be sadly in need at this time. Further care of the mother and investigations will be offered to determine the cause, for possible prevention in another pregnancy.

RESOURCES:

TOMMY'S INFORMATION SERVICE

MISCARRIAGE - INFORMATION AND SUPPORT | TOMMY'S

www.tommys.org/pregnancy-information/pregnancy-complications/baby-loss/miscarriage-information-and-support

No matter when in your pregnancy you miscarry, you may need support to help you come to terms with what's happened. Tommy's is here to help you. You can talk to Tommy's midwife for free, Monday-Friday, 9 am-5 pm. You can call them on 0800 0147 800 or email **midwife@tommys.org**.

SANDS

www.sands.org.uk

Emotional & practical support for anyone affected by the loss of a baby. across the UK

THE MISCARRIAGE ASSOCIATION MID-2ND TRIMESTER LOSS

https://www.miscarriageassociation.org.uk/your-feelings/special-circumstances/late-miscarriage/

Information & support for those who've experienced a late miscarriage. Factsheets & information. Pregnancy loss helpline. Online support.

FOETAL LOSS IN THE WOMB

Very rarely, a baby dies when still in the womb for reasons which may or may not be known.

This can happen at any time up to a full-term pregnancy, and it is easy to imagine the pain, grief and devastation suffered by the parents and family.

After the diagnosis, there will be great shock and distress and time will be allowed for the mother, or couple, to go home, to spend some time together, to make social arrangements and to collect personal items. It will be necessary for the mother to return to the hospital for the baby to be born, usually vaginally, after inducement.

This is a very difficult, emotional event and the staff involved are aware of the special needs and will show every care and compassion.

Most hospitals have a special quiet, private area away from the general, busy departments, where support can be given sensitively, and advice for the later arrangements for baby and any other necessary procedures.

Staff on these units are knowledgeable and specially trained and can put you in touch with all the necessary procedures and help that is available.

You may have religious needs and wish your baby to be blessed. This will be respected and supported by the hospital staff.

RESOURCES:

SUPPORT AFTER BABY LOSS | BEREAVEMENT SUPPORT AND ADVICE

www.sands.org.uk/

Sands, support anyone affected by the death of a baby and works to save babies' lives. We offer support via a helpline, online community, app, local groups and more. across the UK. For everyone. For health professionals. Support for parents. Helpline: 0808 164 3332 / helpline@sands.org.uk

STILLBIRTH

When a baby shows no sign of life immediately after birth it is described as a *still-birth* and can occur without any warning, although it is more usual that warning signs will occur during monitoring as the labour progresses.

There is incredible grief and loss of a child; unimaginable for those of us who have not had personal experience. Nothing anyone can say at this time will soften your pain and you will, understandably, be asking for explanations. It is not always possible to save the baby, for many reasons which need to be investigated and explained later. There may have been a previously undetected birth defect incompatible with life outside the womb.

You will be supported sensitively, and helped by a specialist midwife who will ask you about your wishes, which are very personal to you. The legal requirements will be explained with compassion. There are many issues to deal with at a time when you are in the worst possible position to be making major decisions, but there are many ways to help you, which can be explained at the time.

Appropriate grief counselling will be offered, and all the help and support that is available at this heart-breaking time.

RESOURCES:

STILLBIRTH - **NHS**

https://www.nhs.uk/conditions/stillbirth

Helpline: 0808 164 3332

Sands Helpline - **0808 164 3332**
helpline@sands.org.uk | Sands

www.sands.org.uk/support-you/how-we-offer-support/helpline

The Sands National Helpline provides a safe, confidential place for anyone who has been affected by the death of a baby. Whether your baby died long ago or recently, we are here for you. The telephone helpline is free to call from landlines and mobiles on 0808 164 3332. The helpline team can also be contacted at helpline@sands.org.uk

Cuddlecots: Invention allows parents of stillborn children to spend...

www.independent.co.uk/life-style/health-and-families/cuddlecots-invention-parents-stillborn-children-spend-extra-days-dead-babies-a7664916.html

4 Apr 2017 - Flexmort developed the CuddleCot - a cot that cools the baby and therefore prolongs the amount of time parents can spend with their baby.

BECOMING A PARENT DURING THE RESTRICTIONS OF THE COVID-19 PANDEMIC

The manuscript for this book was written before the Coronavirus Pandemic of 2019, which was a highly contagious virus that had never been experienced before, and the UK lockdown of 23rd March 2020.

The virus was believed to have originated in China in the latter part of 2019 and began to spread worldwide in the early months of 2020. There was a suggestion that wild animals were involved, amongst many other theories.

Little was known of its effects on humans, except that it attacked the lungs and, from there, to other organs in the body, depleting them of oxygen and often requiring intensive care treatment, sometimes on life-supporting ventilators.

The virus lives for long periods on surfaces, so thorough and regular hand cleaning became an important preventative measure. Keeping to social distances of 2 metres was also advised to prevent passing the virus infection via droplets in the air. People were advised not to touch their faces.

In the earlier stages of the spread, the death rate was high, mostly affecting the aged and those with underlying health issues. Pregnant women were amongst those who required 'shielding' by staying in their homes, isolating themselves from outsiders and limiting their antenatal appointments to essential-only contact with hospital or clinic staff; they also had to shield themselves with personal protection equipment (PPE). This meant covering their faces with face masks and whole-face transparent plastic visors and wearing disposable gloves, protective, waterproof outer garments and outer shoe coverings.

Husbands and partners were unable to attend antenatal appointments or procedures such as the scans to monitor the baby's growth etc. During the birth, the birth partner could only stay for established labour until the birth, and postnatal visits were not permitted.

After birth, health checks by midwives and health visitors were limited to phone calls and only essential home visits to observe mother and baby were allowed.

At the end of March 2020, the UK government imposed a 'lockdown', which meant all household members had to stay in their homes, only going out for essential items such as food and medical supplies. Keyworkers were allowed to work and only shops selling essential supplies were allowed to open. Schools were closed and children had home-schooling as far as was possible. Food and other supplies could be left outside the homes of vulnerable people by someone keeping a safe distance. It became a strange, empty world outside homes.

This was an unprecedented experience for everybody, and parents-to-be had their own unique inconveniences and anxieties during these arrangements.

There is always a silver lining to all dark clouds, however, and in many ways, some people found advantages in this new way of life. Television and the internet became a lifeline for those people locked in their homes.

There is anecdotal information that newborn babies are regaining their birth weight at five days when the expected time is ten days. Could this be due to the lack of disturbance from visitors and check-ups by professionals that have allowed the parents peace, and quiet to spend more time alone to bond and care for their baby?

Postpartum Recovery in a Pandemic | Healthy Mama Hacks

https://healthymamahacks.net/postpartum-recovery-in-a-pandemic/#:~:text=Although%20it%E2%80%99s%20completely%20normal%20for%20newborns%20to%20lose,care%29%20are%20returning%20to%20birth%20weight%20much%20sooner.

Surprisingly, other anecdotal reports suggest a reduction in the incidence of babies being born preterm during the lockdown. Could this be because pregnant women had a less stressful life, not having to travel to work or other activities and generally having more rest and less anxiety, despite the general anxiety of all the unknowns and disruptions to everyday life?

No doubt, much research will take place and lessons learnt for future generations to come, so some good could come out of a bad situation.

A REDUCTION IN PREMATURE BIRTHS DURING COVID-19

https://www.rcm.org.uk/news-views/rcm-opinion/2020/a-reduction-in-premature-births-during-covid-19/

24/07/2020 A remarkable reduction in premature birth has been found in two studies. Although neither has yet been published in peer-reviewed journals, the findings from Ireland and Denmark are receiving plenty of interest. The findings of both studies show a dramatic reduction in the numbers of premature births during the lockdown.

SOME PARENTS EXPERIENCES OF SURVIVING BIRTH DURING THE COVID-19 PANDEMIC AND LOCKDOWN OF 2020

This book is about looking forward to birth with all the support and help from the professionals involved in providing care throughout the pregnancy, birth and caring for the newborn.

The stories below are from parents experiencing this hugely emotional and life-changing period, planning and looking forward to all the facilities and caring culture we have become used to and take for granted.

Because of the restrictions necessarily imposed, the reality was far from what they expected, and the suddenness of the onset added to the anxiety.

It is to be hoped that with all that has been learnt about this Covid-19 virus, restrictions will be lifted as more testing can be carried out and a safe vaccine is found for our protection. We look forward to a return to 'normal' soon.

The stories below need to be told as a historical record of how this dangerous virus forced changes in the culture of giving birth in the UK to the detriment and, strangely, to the benefit of some.

KATE AND FREDDY BECAME THE PARENTS OF A BABY GIRL, PRIMROSE ELIZABETH, ON 29TH MAY 2020

They have described how the restrictions of lockdown and their antenatal, birth and postnatal experiences affected their lives and the memory of becoming first-time parents at this time in our history.

KATE

…having my first child during a global pandemic was not an experience I will forget in a hurry.

I had imagined having a relaxing few weeks leading up to my due date having afternoon tea with my friends and shopping to buy baby clothes with my mum. Instead, I was stuck inside my house on lockdown for the last 3 months of my pregnancy, unable to leave my house or welcome any visitors or guests.'

Lockdown didn't just mean that I couldn't leave the house, it also meant that the NHS antenatal classes that I had expected to attend had been cancelled, a lot of my routine antenatal appointments had been cancelled, and the ones I could go to, I had to go alone.

Although the NHS antenatal classes had been cancelled I was very lucky in that Maureen Gannon volunteered her experience and knowledge to help mothers to be in my position by offering them free online classes to help provide some guidance about giving birth. I found her advice extremely helpful and comforting; without her help, I would have been lost with a lot of the things that ended up happening. Similarly, this book has been a very helpful and informative guide for myself and my husband.

Kate had a relatively straightforward pregnancy, but at thirty-seven weeks, for obstetric reasons, she required hospital procedures, over a few days and while she was alone, which eventually led to the birth of her baby.

The hardest part for Kate:'...was having to attend these scans and appointments alone, without the support and comfort of my husband'.

...it meant everything was on my shoulders; I couldn't share the pressure with my husband as would have been routine. In addition, my husband couldn't see our baby on the screen as I could, and he couldn't ask the doctor about any concerns or questions he may have had (or I had forgotten to ask in the anx.)

Kate found the midwives pleasant and, although during her two and a half days in hospital she bonded with the other new mothers, she was lonely with a newborn baby, which was not what she expected at all. Sadly this was the medical science and advice to save lives and slow down the spread of a deadly new virus.

KATE

On the bright side - I have a very lovely, healthy, happy baby. So, it seems to have been a means to an end! And I count it all as character building.

Angharad and Luke became the parents of baby Owain on 7th June 2020

Pregnancy and post-birth story

When we found out back in early October that we were expecting our first child we could have never imagined how different the world would be when our due date arrived! Luckily the whole pregnancy had gone very smoothly but when Boris made his announcement in March that pregnant women were being placed in the high-risk group everything suddenly felt very scary.
Two days later and I was sent home from work with no plan to return before my maternity leave started. There was no big fair well, no baby shower and no pre-baby outings once lockdown commenced. Being able to work from home did have its positives though, I didn't have to worry about finding shoes to fit, or commute to work every day whilst heavily pregnant!!

Two days after my due date contractions started which continued for 40 hours until a new midwife who had just started her shift told me whilst doing a routine check that something didn't feel right...my baby was brow presentation and after trying and failing to get him to move with a hormone drip an emergency c section was needed. Luckily Luke was able to be in theatre for the whole thing and my beautiful boy entered the world!

The hardest part of covid for me and Luke was knowing that once I and baby Owain entered the recovery ward we wouldn't be able to see him again until we left, not even for visiting! From this point onwards I was desperate for us to come home as soon as possible. Not being able to have any visitors was so hard, after 2 nights we were finally allowed to come home. The struggles of covid didn't end there, home visits from midwives and health visitors were all banned, and after major surgery, the last thing I wanted was to be backwards and forwards to the appointments every couple of days. Partners were also banned so this was another aspect that unfortunately, Luke couldn't be a part of. Visits from people were from the doorway only for the first few weeks, they were short but sweet although going backwards and forwards to the door whilst juggling a newborn and holding my stitches was in a way harder, luckily for me, Luke took charge of all nappy changes and my mum dropped off endless meals to stop us going hungry.

As the weeks went by and restrictions started to ease things have gotten easier and easier but baby Owain is still yet to be held by family or friends without a face mask. Having a baby during covid has had some big positives and big negatives but we will never forget bringing our perfect baby boy into the world in the middle of a pandemic which one day he will learn about in school.

Charlotte and Nick had a baby boy, Milo, on 29th January 2020

Our experiences of a 'lockdown baby

Our baby was born on 29th January, luckily for us, COVID-19 wasn't really on our radar, we were blessed with a great birth, baby Milo took to feeding well and we had a lovely few weeks at home together before my husband went back to work.

I had actually put our family into 'lockdown' the week before Boris, with the emerging news and data I was scared for our tiny baby, his little immune system not yet developed, how would he cope with the virus? How would we be able to look after the children effectively if we caught it? My husband was able to work from home easily, so I pulled our 3-year-old out of preschool and ensured we had a food delivery slot booked!

I remember a nervous excitement at it all which soon wore very thin as the days and weeks followed. We still had to leave the house for Milos jabs, it was before masks became a necessity and I was really worried about going, the visit was fine although I couldn't take his red book, pushchair or his sibling. I still cried when I got home- so scared that I had put our baby, myself and our little family in danger. It's my job to keep my babies safe and I really felt for the first few months I couldn't do that, the virus was so unknown, death and infection rates were rising and there was absolutely nothing I could do. I felt so guilty that Milo did not have the same start in life that his brother Warren did, what long term effects will this have on my boys? What sort of world have we bought them into? I felt angry that others were not taking it seriously and still living their lives as normal, silently spreading this virus that has taken away our freedom. I had to stop watching and reading the news, it made me cry and I couldn't let the boys be aware of what was happening, we stayed in our little bubble and shut out the rest of the world.

In regards to being in lockdown, it certainly had its pros and cons for our family, my husband has been able to spend so much time with our boys, he's been able to get up in the morning with our three-year-old for breakfast so I could catch up on sleep with the baby, he's been joining us for lunch, cooking dinner and helping out with poo explosions! He would have missed so many 'firsts' had he been at work.

I also think breastfeeding has gone so well because it has been on-demand, with no fear of needing to cover up, find somewhere suitable to sit or rushing around to playgroup or the shops and the baby having to wait.

Aside from the pandemic itself the cons of lockdown have been the lack of social interaction for our boys, Milo has missed out on meeting and seeing family and friends and they have missed his baby stage, missed those curled up squishy cuddles, those first smiles and coos and that beautiful milky baby smell that you wish you could bottle! Even now we are out and about he does not have the interaction from strangers in the queues at the supermarket, everyone is anonymous with their masks covering silly faces and generous smiles everyone normally has for little babies.

My three-year-old Warren has struggled with his behaviour and emotions, without the structure of preschool and social interactions we have had lots of meltdowns and pushing of boundaries, how much do we let slide because it must be hard for him to deal with?

Aside from the terrible side it has made me appreciate family and friends, the benefits of a village when raising children has been missed, I cannot wait until we can get back to 'normal', hug people without a second thought, pass the baby to someone else when it all gets too much and see my three-year-old have cuddles with his grandparents.

I feel guilty for thinking 2020 has been a terrible year, it's the year we completed our family with our beautiful, bright boy, we are hoping he will never remember this strange start to life although we are sure he will be known as a 'lockdown baby' forever!

EMMA AND SCOTT HAD A BABY BOY, DOMINIC, ON THE 20TH MARCH 2020, THREE DAYS BEFORE LOCKDOWN WHICH WAS ON 23RD MARCH.

EMMA

My thoughts and feelings on having a lockdown baby.

It has been an emotional time having my first child at the beginning of covid lockdown. I gave birth by caesarean 3 days before we were out into lockdown so that in itself was scary. I was excited for my parents to meet their first grandchild but only I was allowed into the ward which was very upsetting for all of us.

I was so excited to get home and for all our family and friends to meet him which sadly didn't happen. Then to be stuck in for 4 months with only being allowed out for daily exercise and appointments really didn't help, I was contacted by the health visitor weekly, to begin with, by telephone which was ok but it didn't help me with breastfeeding.

I had 6 weeks of painful feeding and using a breast pump. As we have had no groups happening I struggled with feeding issues which I think could have helped me very much. As for other groups to meet other mums would have been very nice. My family have been amazing though they have helped me so much.

I feel like I have missed out on days out and time with my baby due to covid I wish they could have extended paid maternity leave so I could have more time but sadly they didn't which means I have to go back to work in January. Xxx

Chloe Mo and Andrew had a baby girl, Hawaii Blossom Mai, on the 1st February 2020

Whilst 2020 has been a distressing time for us all, it has been ultimately distressing/challenging for mothers expecting or who have just given birth. I became a first time mum to a beautiful baby girl just before the coronavirus outbreak began.

For me, I experienced what we call the 'normal' labour experience and aftercare, as opposed to what care other mothers are, or having to experience now. Whilst, I was lucky enough to receive the initial aftercare from the community midwives/health visitor for the first three weeks it all stopped after that.

A few days before my 5 weeks old was taken to hospital with a 40-degree temperature and a heart rate of 200 I had a phone call from the health visitor stating that home visits were stopped because of the coronavirus. I had only met her a handful of times before that. I felt very alone, anxious and scared being blue lighted from our local GP to the hospital where she underwent numerous tests including the covid 19 and lumbar puncture, which thankfully came back all clear, everything just felt so surreal. That was the last time I or her had any interaction with all health professionals, excluding the 2 minute appointments for her standard injections. Due to this pandemic.

My daughter has been stripped of any normal interaction with friends, family and other babies. My daughter is now 7 months old and has severe separation anxiety. I am full of fear that if I take her out she or I may catch something although restrictions have been lifted and the first thing I do when I get home is check her temperature. Ultimately, the one thing I wanted to do was show her off to the world, being a new mum, but that hasn't been able to happen due to this pandemic. It has been very difficult.

I'm currently 21 weeks pregnant with my second child and the antenatal care I'm receiving now is completely different. All consultations have been done over the phone, and I haven't actually seen my midwife. I've also had to attend scans/ hospital appointments all on my own. Of course, we don't know when all of this will end but it's very daunting not knowing what will be this time.

HOLLIE AND LUKE HAD A BABY DAUGHTER, OLIVIA, SISTER TO AMELIA, BORN ON THE 25TH APRIL 2020

Giving birth in a pandemic almost felt surreal. Those first moments that you imagine when pregnant, all taken away from you. My innocent and perfect baby had to meet her grandparents through a window and waited months until that first cuddle. The guilt as a parent, of feeling like you, haven't been able to enjoy this special time as much because you're scared of taking your baby even outside the front door, constantly watching to make sure nobody is approaching, rather than watching those little blue eyes staring up at you from the pram.

It has been a very lonely journey as a second-time new mum, without the support of groups and other mums, but having quality time with my newborn and her big sister made all this worth it. Spending those first few months getting used to life as a new family without interruption only made our bond stronger! Our baby is definitely the light at the end of the rainbow.

All the parents have given their permission for their stories to be published.

Acknowledgements

As a mature student of midwifery, I have brought my personal experiences of childbirth to this book. Plus, I have always been a follower of the late Grantly Dick-Read. His book, *Childbirth Without Fear*, is still being published and his teachings greatly influenced me during the births of my babies, during my training and later within my midwifery practice.

I have been greatly influenced by Frédérick Leboyer (deceased 2017), who, in his book *Birth Without Violence*, advocated birth without loud noises, shouting, banging and clanging of hospital trolleys. But especially without the horrific practice of previous times, such as that of holding the baby upside-down by its feet and smacking its bottom to stimulate breathing. Thankfully, I have never witnessed such abuse of a newborn.

Instead, Leboyer advocated a quiet, calm atmosphere with dim lights, gentle handling of the baby as it is born, and, at the appropriate time, immersing the baby in deep, warm water to simulate the warm, moist conditions of the womb.

As a midwife, I endeavoured to induce calmness in the labour room according to his teachings - as much as hospital protocol would allow - and I teach his methods in my Hypnobirthing Antenatal Classes. Frédéric Leboyer's books are still being published too.

Michel Odent, the founder of the *Primal Health Research Centre*, London, prolific author of numerous books promoting natural birth and known pioneer of water birth, encourages women to listen to their bodies, to give birth in quiet, calm surroundings with no intervention unless absolutely necessary, promotes calmness, giving the mother privacy, with as little interruption as possible, thus allowing her to relax and follow her own instincts.

I have attended many of his lectures, been a follower of his teachings throughout my career and have completed his four-day doula course in London. He is a man of many talents, a brilliant researcher and passionate about mother and baby welfare.

I am grateful to the late Sheila Kitzinger, social anthropologist and author supporting women in childbirth. In her book, *The New Experience of Childbirth*, she described the procedure of episiotomy (then routine at every birth) as unkind and mostly unnecessary, which changed the protocols midwives were obliged to follow and allowed us to use our discretion. This marked a major change in the management of birth to the benefit of many thousands of women.

Later, I attended a one-day conference on gentle caesarean births, with Jenny Smith, founder of the *Jentle Birth Foundation*, and Michel Odent. I was greatly impressed by the dedication of many birth professionals who are eager to make a planned caesarean birth be as lovely an experience as natural birth. It can be done if enough people want to make it happen.

One of the many study days I attended was with Andrea Robertson, author of *The Midwife Companion* and other books, and it was there I met Jean Sutton, who wrote *Let Birth be Born Again* but who is now retired in her home country of New Zealand.

Jean comes from a farming and engineering background as well as midwifery. She studied the anatomy of the maternal pelvis and its relationship to the foetal head, comparing them with old midwifery textbooks. Looking at it from an engineering perspective, she came up with the concept of *Optimal Foetal Positioning* - rewriting the anatomy books. It was the first time I had heard of the amazing *Rhombus of Michaelis* and its importance at the point of birth. Something else I did not learn in my midwifery training...

With Jean's permission, I have used some of the contents of her book to promote this concept of natural birth, helping to educate women to know exactly what is happening to their bodies when the miracle of birth unfolds. I thank Jean for all that I have learnt from her amazing knowledge, and for the chance to use it in my antenatal/hypnobirthing classes, as well as in this book. Knowledge is power.

I first heard Sally Inch lecturing on *The Cascade of Intervention* in Cardiff, and it was fascinating. It all made sense, so I have incorporated this message in my classes and this book. Sally is another pioneer of natural birth, and her books have spread the word worldwide, making people think before they begin intervention as it can trigger the cascade of intervention that may follow.

I would also like to thank Laura Bagnall, Illustrator, for clearly showing the different muscles of the uterus, the procedures for epidural and spinal anaesthesia, and the waves of contraction of the womb during labour through her line drawings. Her talent is also expressed in her artistic contribution to my book, *The Survival Guide for New Parents*.

Last but certainly not least, as a community midwife in a rural area of Somerset, I met Hannah Giffard, an art student, and Keith Tutt, a university graduate, living in a lovely little cottage, pregnant and requesting a home birth. They had the most wonderful philosophy and were lovingly anticipating the birth of their baby. Never was a baby more wanted or more lovingly prepared for.

Hannah and Keith wanted a natural birth, without pain relief or other medication. One with a Leboyer-style quiet and calm atmosphere, with dim lighting, for baby to be immersed in deep, warm water after the birth, then wrapped in a beautiful soft blanket without any other clothes – not even a nappy.

During the hours of labour, we developed a rapport and a friendship that has survived to this day. Baby Luke, was born, immersed in deep, warm water, breastfed and peacefully placed in his cot, wrapped in his beautiful soft blanket. We celebrated his arrival with small pots of Saki, especially saved for the occasion. Two years later, I was privileged to be in attendance when baby, Joe, was born in the same calm and loving way.

Hannah and Keith taught me things about birth that I never learnt during my midwifery training, but it shaped me as a midwife and deepened my understanding of the need for respect and tranquillity during the birthing process.

A big thank you to Ann Brady, Mentoring Writers, for rescuing me and taking me under her wing when my book was in the doldrums, and publication was fraught with never ending delays. She gave me hope, and the reality of publication at last. I am grateful.

BIBLIOGRAPHY

SUTTON, Jean, Let Birth be Born Again. Birth Concepts. UK.

Some text and illustration, The Birthing Partnership course, have been sourced from Jean Sutton's book; her permission has been obtained to use the excerpts. Highly recommended to all parents-to-be.

BRAZELTON, T, Berry, MD and NUGENT, J. Kevin. (1995) Neonatal Behaviour Assessment Scale. Cambridge University Press.

FOSTER, Rachel, LONGTON, Carrie and ROBERTS, Justine. Mums on Babies: Trade secrets from the real experts. Cassell Illustrated. www.mumsnet.com

DICK-READ, Grantly. (1958) Childbirth without Fear. William Heinemann Medical Books Ltd.

GERHARDT, Sue. (2009) Why Love Matters: How affection shapes a baby's brain. Routledge Publishers

GORDON, Yehudi. (2002) Birth and Beyond. Vermillion.

JOHNSTON, Peter G. B. (1998) The New-born Child. Churchill Livingstone.
KLAUS, Marshall H. and KLAUS, Phyllis H. (1999) Your Amazing New-born. Perseus Books, Cambridge, Massachusetts.

LEBOYER, Frédérick. (1975) Birth without Violence. Fletcher & Son Ltd., Norwich.

MOTHA, Dr Gowri. (2004) Gentle Birth Method. Harper Collins.

NILSSON, Lennart. (1990) A Child Is Born. Doubleday.

ODENT, Michel. (2004) Primal Health Research Centre, London.

ODENT, Michel. (2013) Childbirth and the future of homo sapiens. Paperback - November 7, 2013.

Birth under water - Michel Odent - Active Birth Pools 12 Oct 2016

KITZINGER, Sheila. New Experience of Childbirth. 2004

ROBERTSON, Andrea. Making Birth Easier. Allen and Unwin.
ROBERTSON, Andrea. Preparing for Birth: Mothers. Birth International.

Highly recommended:

ROBERTSON, Andrea. Preparing for Birth: Fathers. Birth International.

Highly recommended as very little reading for fathers is available:

SMALL, Meredith. (1999) Our Babies Ourselves. Anchor Books, Doubleday.

TEW, Marjorie. (1990) Safer Childbirth. Chapman and Hall.

VERNY, Dr Thomas with KELLY, John. The Secret Life of the Unborn Child. Sphere Books Limited.

GANNON, Maureen. (2017) The Survival Guide for New Parents. Wordcatcher Publishing.

GANNON, Maureen. The Survival Guide for New Parents. Updated 2nd edition (2021)

KNOWLES, Rosie. (2016) Why Baby Wearing Matters. Pinter & Martin Ltd.

Lightning Source UK Ltd.
Milton Keynes UK
UKHW021153061221
395181UK00007B/360

9 780993 112966